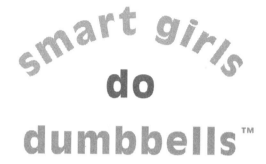

smart girls
do
dumbbells™

judith sherman-wolin

ACSM HEALTH FITNESS INSTRUCTOR® • NSCA CERTIFIED PERSONAL TRAINER

smart girls
do
dumbbells™

RIVERHEAD BOOKS

New York

Most Riverhead Books are available at special quantity discounts for bulk purchases for sales promotions, premiums, fund-raising, or educational use. Special books, or book excerpts, can also be created to fit specific needs.

For details, write: Special Markets, The Berkley Publishing Group, 375 Hudson Street, New York, New York 10014.

THE BERKLEY PUBLISHING GROUP
Published by the Penguin Group
Penguin Group (USA) Inc.
375 Hudson Street, New York, New York 10014, USA
Penguin Group (Canada), 10 Alcorn Avenue, Toronto, Ontario M4V 3B2, Canada
(a division of Pearson Penguin Canada Inc.)
Penguin Books Ltd., 80 Strand, London WC2R 0RL, England
Penguin Group Ireland, 25 St. Stephen's Green, Dublin 2, Ireland (a division of Penguin Books Ltd.)
Penguin Group (Australia), 250 Camberwell Road, Camberwell, Victoria 3124, Australia
(a division of Pearson Australia Group Pty. Ltd.)
Penguin Books India Pvt. Ltd., 11 Community Centre, Panchsheel Park, New Delhi—110 017, India
Penguin Group (NZ), Cnr. Airborne and Rosedale Roads, Albany, Auckland 1310, New Zealand
(a division of Pearson New Zealand Ltd.)
Penguin Books (South Africa) (Pty.) Ltd., 24 Sturdee Avenue, Rosebank, Johannesburg 2196,
South Africa

Penguin Books Ltd., Registered Offices: 80 Strand, London WC2R 0RL, England

Every effort has been made to ensure that the information contained in this book is complete and accurate. However, neither the publisher nor the author is engaged in rendering professional advice or services to the individual reader. The ideas, procedures, and suggestions contained in this book are not intended as a substitute for consulting with your physician. All matters regarding your health require medical supervision. Neither the author nor the publisher shall be liable or responsible for any loss, injury, or damage allegedly arising from any information or suggestions in this book.

PRINTING HISTORY
First Riverhead trade paperback edition: April 2004

Library of Congress Cataloging-in-Publication Data

Sherman-Wolin, Judith.
    Smart girls do dumbbells / Judith Sherman-Wolin.–1st ed.
        p. cm.
    ISBN 1-57322-386-7
    1. Bodybuilding for women.   I. Title.

GV546.6.W64S465   2004
613.7'1'082–dc22
                                           2003070433

PRINTED IN THE UNITED STATES OF AMERICA

14 13 12 11 10 9 8 7 6 5

For my children, Samantha and Bennett, the prides of my heart.

contents

foreword

I am a great proponent of exercise. It is one of the best ways to maintain a healthy body and healthy weight once you have lost weight. Aerobic exercise by itself does not always result in effective weight loss; that's why it is so important to include a dumbbell workout in your routine. Once you start doing your dumbbell program regularly, you will be hooked. The blood levels of a hormone called endorphin will rise in anticipation of your exercise session and you will feel deprived if you don't get a chance to exercise.

In *Smart Girls Do Dumbbells* you will learn practical ways to use dumbbells. I use them every morning at home, exercising different muscle groups. I find them at hotels or local gyms when I travel. I couldn't live without my regular dumbbell exercises. I like to say that exercise is no longer an option but a necessity given our almost totally sedentary lifestyles and the high fat, high sugar, and high starch food environment. Today over 60 percent of Americans are overweight as the result of too little exercise and too much food. And, while it is safe to exercise while dieting, you should always consult your physician before starting any exercise program.

Judith Sherman-Wolin has done a great job in describing 30 Dumbbell Exercise Recipes in a simple and easy-to-understand fashion and designing a 30-Day Program you can do regularly at home or in a gym without becoming bored. You will learn how to exercise to maximize your results by building muscle to increase the number of calories you are burning. In fact, every pound of muscle burns fourteen calories per day and so ten additional pounds of muscle means that you will lose an additional one-third of a pound on a diet or be able to eat 140 calories more and maintain your weight.

Building muscle mass by following the well-designed program described in *Smart Girls Do Dumbbells* can also improve your posture and self-esteem, and exercise on a regular basis can also help reduce your stress. In my view, it is the only healthy addiction.

David Heber, M.D., Ph.D.
Professor of Medicine and Public Health,
David Geffen School of Medicine at UCLA
Director, UCLA Center for Human Nutrition

acknowledgments

A special thank-you and an immense debt of gratitude goes to Dr. David Heber, who gave me a home at the UCLA Center for Human Nutrition and shared his patients with me. His dedication to nutritional science and public health is defining the future of health care in this country. It is an honor to work in the light of such brilliance each day.

Deep appreciation goes to my creative and supportive editors at Riverhead Books. Amy Hertz, who gave me one of the most wonderful birthday presents ever, when a year ago I picked up the phone and the first words she said to me were, "I love your book." Erin Moore, a unique being . . . a bodybuilder and an editor, who embraced my message and helped tremendously in fine-tuning it. Janie Fleming and Marc Haeringer for their continuous guidance, especially ushering me through the prickly process of production.

A huge thank-you to Aviva Covitz, client and friend, who played a pivotal role in helping this book become a reality.

And a very special thank-you goes to my creative soul sister Lori Milken. She was the first person to read the pages of my book, give me invaluable editing suggestions and provide constant encouragement during our monthly creative meetings. A talented writer in her own right and one of the most remarkable women I know.

To Nancy and Howard Marks, I don't know where to begin. The most generous and dearest of friends, together and individually, they have been constant wellsprings of love, friendship, and unconditional support. Howard, valued advisor and counselor, who never fails to take a call or answer a question. As brilliant in his knowledge of art and antiques as he is in the art of finance, his advice has been invaluable to my well-being and that of my children. And Nancy, who sets the standard of beauty, richness of heart, and incomparable grace . . . anyone fortunate enough to spend even the briefest moment with her, walks away knowing they have been in the presence of an extraordinary woman.

To my friends, walking partners, and safety nets: Ellen Sandler, Carole Robbins, Wendy Woskoff, Jill Chozen, Katherine Nouri Houghes, Hillari Koppelman and Judy Hirsch, each one an amazing and accomplished woman with whom I have shared hours and hours, years and decades of walks and talks, laughter and tears, tragedies and triumphs, good friends all . . . and all deeply loved.

A kiss and a hug go to my dear childhood friend Philip Gary Miller, who had absolutely nothing to do with this book, but who held my hand down some rocky roads and wouldn't let me fall. His friendship is a valued treasure I hold close to my heart always.

To my longtime training partner Mitchell Ohlbaum, who taught me the gym is not only a place in which to build muscle, but a place to build friendship. If not for Mitchy, many 5 A.M. workouts would not have been nearly so tolerable, nor hilarious.

I am also extremely grateful to the patients I have worked with over the last six years at the UCLA Center for Human Nutrition and the RFO Program, many of whom have faced tremendous personal battles and crushing health issues. Each day, I am allowed the privilege of teaching them how to build muscle and strength, and in return, they teach me about courage, faith, and the remarkable stamina of the human spirit.

And finally, in memory of Ronald Wolin, brilliant artist and adored father, who shared with me the greatest gifts either of us could ever have hoped for or imagined, our cherished and amazing children, Samantha and Bennett.

introduction

Everyone knows that a well-made body lasts a long time.
— COLLETTE

I have been a practicing health-fitness educator and journalist for almost two decades. In my private practice, and working with patients at the UCLA Center for Human Nutrition, I have witnessed remarkable changes. I work with women who have lost more than a hundred pounds. I work with women who couldn't lift a one-pound dumbbell and now lift fifteen pounds. I work with women who have increased their bone density, flexibility, and muscle mass and lowered their blood sugar, blood pressure, and risk for cardiovascular disease, type 2 diabetes, and some cancers. They come to me with different goals, capabilities, and tolerance for exercise, but the one element all these women share in common is this: *Not one ever regrets the time she spends learning how to build a leaner, healthier, more beautiful body.*

If you have a true desire and honest commitment to follow the exercise techniques and the 30-Day Program described in this book, you will see positive results, *guaranteed.*

You will:

- Build a healthier body composition
- Have a leaner body

- Burn more calories daily
- Have stronger joints and ligaments
- Protect and build your bones
- Create flatter abdominals and increase core strength
- Gain physical strength and personal power
- Lower your risk for heart disease, some types of cancer, high blood pressure, diabetes, and bone loss
- Look and feel better
- Be happier with yourself and take pride in your accomplishments

I am not going to lie to you—exercise isn't always easy and it isn't always fun. Some fitness experts try to gimmick it up and gloss it over, but the bottom line is: It's work. It doesn't always come naturally or easily. Sometimes it takes forced commitment and overcoming your prejudices about the time and effort involved, but as you will discover, it pays off big time! As I tell the women I work with every day who do the work and reap the rewards, I can promise you this: You will learn how to perform the dumbbell exercises—*properly*. You will realize results—*steadily*. You will learn valuable techniques for sticking with your exercise program—*consistently*. At the end of the day, you might even learn to enjoy your dumbbell workouts (*hopefully!*).

Maintaining a strong body is not only health promoting, it can be healing. It is the elusive Fountain of Youth. It keeps you vital and vibrant. As I said in the beginning, it isn't always easy or fun, but it is always worth the effort. *Always.*

Smart Girls Do Dumbbells is, yes, primarily a book teaching you the importance and beauty of muscle, how to do the dumbbell exercises correctly, and how to become a lifelong exerciser by getting into the Exercise Success Triad. Equally important, however, is learning to embrace a life of courage and confidence. You will find that as you grow muscle, you grow personal power.

Our bodies need food to survive. Our bodies need exercise to survive . . . *beautifully.*

For all these reasons, and probably some reasons of your own . . . *Smart Girls Do Dumbbells.*

· 1 ·

why muscle
matters

What if I told you there is a natural, seemingly magical way for you to burn a greater number of calories without moving? Well, there is. It's called muscle!

Muscle is a metabolically active tissue. That means it burns around 14 calories per pound per twenty-four-hour period. There are some estimates that fat burns only around 3 calories per pound. So the more muscle you have, the more calories you burn daily. Muscle does not age-discriminate, either. If you want to increase your muscle mass so you can burn more calories, you have only to follow the techniques and training protocols outlined in this book. Muscle will grow. Calories will burn. Fat will stay off.

I'd like to dispel one myth immediately: You do not have enough of the right hormones to end up looking muscle-bound. I hear this concern expressed constantly: "I don't want to end up looking like Arnold Schwarzenegger." I assure you, if you're not tinkering with your hormones by taking anabolic steroids or performance-enhancing drugs and you're training according to the program in this book, you will not build bulky, manly muscles.

But you also have to keep your body type in mind. Some women naturally carry more muscle and develop it faster and more easily than others.

If that is you, you need to follow a training program (which I will talk about later) that will allow you to sculpt your body the way you want without becoming overly muscular.

· muscle burns calories, but that's not all! ·

Muscle is a twenty-four-hour furnace, allowing you to burn more calories *even at rest.* Muscle is the body's major metabolic booster. The famous "yo-yo" dieting syndrome is a result of muscle loss—if you diet without exercising, you lose muscle along with fat and the loss of muscle tissue translates into a slowdown—sometimes a shutdown—of your metabolism. Eating less will help you lose weight, but building muscle will help you keep it off.

· muscle-building promotes bone health ·

We tend to think of our bones as hard, almost lifeless structures that keep us upright, fixed, and solid. Nothing could be further from the truth. Bone is a constantly changing tissue: growing, diminishing, and remodeling.

Women's bones are much more vulnerable than men's. We stop building bone between the ages of thirty and thirty-five, and after menopause we start losing bone. It is estimated that four to six million women in the United States have osteoporosis—characterized by low bone density and weakening of the infrastructure of the bones. An additional thirteen to seventeen million have low bone density (osteopenia), primarily at the hip.

As women age, bone health is compromised. But the good news is you are in charge of your bones.

In addition to taking calcium supplements, one of the recommended preventative interventions is exercise! Many health organizations are currently conducting studies on exactly how and to what extent exercise impacts bone health. All of the answers aren't in, but we do know this: A regular, ongoing program of weight-bearing and weight-resistance exercises is a key strategy for preventing and curtailing weakening and diminishing bones.

I am frequently asked the difference between weight-bearing and weight-resistance exercise.

Weight-bearing exercises are any activities in which you carry your own weight through space, your body opposing gravity. Jogging, walking, running, stair-stepping, dancing, and sports such as soccer and basketball are all examples of weight-bearing exercises.

Weight-resistance exercises use resistance mechanisms, such as dumbbells, that place additional loads on your muscles and bones besides your own body weight. *Weight training* and *weight lifting* are other commonly used terms.

Even though they are good calorie burners, swimming and biking are not weight-bearing exercises. So if you love to swim or bike—great! Don't stop those activities, just add in the dumbbells to help protect and build your bones.

· muscle is an antiaging tissue ·

You want to look and feel young for as long as possible? Muscle. You want to move as fluidly as you did in your youth? Muscle. You want to be strong as long as possible? Muscle. It's all about muscle. You can have plastic surgery from head to toe and slather on all the antiaging creams and youth-promoting lotions you can get your hands on, but none will help—none—if your body is physically weak.

Our bodies lose muscle throughout the aging process. Our muscle mass starts declining at around the age of twenty-five (unless we exercise). We lose about 4 percent per decade starting from the age of twenty-five through age fifty, and about 10 percent per decade thereafter. But it is not true that there's no retrieving it. Current research reveals that muscle responds to resistance training and it does not care how old you are.

According to a study that appeared in *The Physician and Sports Medicine,*

Dr. Joseph Buckwalter reports, "There is growing evidence that training of sufficient intensity can increase strength as effectively in older individuals as younger ones."

What muscle really doesn't like is *not being used*.

Building muscle through exercise also combats the aging process by keeping our bodies and joints strong and functional. We look old when we move sluggishly, when our joints hurt and we have limited range of motion, regardless of our chronological age.

Muscle is a better camouflage for body flaws than wearing black. The important point to understand about muscle is that it is a compact tissue, heavier in composition than fat. So even though it may weigh a bit more, it looks a lot less. As you build muscle and lose fat you might be surprised to find the scale doesn't always reflect a big number decrease but that's okay . . . the muscle you're growing makes a more beautiful, firmer, healthier-looking and feeling body.

Imagine this scenario: You see someone hunched over who can barely walk. You hear her complaining about her aches and pains. Every time she gets up from a chair she moans a bit. Maybe this is an old person or maybe it's a young person with an old back. You'd be surprised how similar they look. Physical weakness looks like aging, regardless of how old the sufferer is.

· muscle helps create
a healthier body ·

Muscle built through exercise has profound physiologic and metabolic benefits. In addition to its high-caloric burn, muscle-building exercise helps remove sugar from the bloodstream and create a body lower in fat. These are important factors in controlling and preventing heart disease, the number one killer of both men and women in the United States, and type 2 diabetes, which is one of the fastest-growing diseases in our country today.

An article appearing in the American Heart Association's journal, *Circulation*, concluded, "Mild to moderate resistance training can provide an effective method for improving muscular strength and endurance, preventing and managing a variety of chronic medical conditions, modifying coronary risk factor, and enhancing psychosocial well-being."

And according to the largest study ever conducted on type 2 diabetes by the National Institutes of Health, this disease can be significantly curtailed through exercise as well as diet. As reported in the *New York Times* when the study results were announced, "Exercise and diet were so effective that the researchers ended their work a year early."

Additionally, muscle helps keep joints strong. Loss of joint range of motion is another sign of aging. Dumbbells provide resistance against muscles, which keeps the ligaments strong. Strong joints also help with allover alignment so your body is less at risk for injury, whether you are performing everyday tasks or participating in a triathlon.

· muscle is empowering ·

Men have always known, ever since they emerged from the primordial sludge, that muscle has intrinsic value far beyond physiologic attributes. Women, we of the "gatherer" gender, are evolutionary latecomers to the power party. I once interviewed several dozen men on the subject of muscle. "What does it mean to you?" I asked. The response was universal: Muscle is power. It means strength and sexuality. Men crave muscle because it gives them a profound sense of control over their lives. I don't know about you, dear readers, but I want control over my life! I want strength and power and to be sexually appealing, too. If muscle is the magic tissue that's going to do that for me, may I have some, please?

If there was ever a question in your mind why *smart girls do dumbbells*, now you have plenty of evidence. The muscle you build doing the dumbbell exercises you'll learn in this book is a relentless calorie consumer. It's always on the job; it never goes on vacations or holidays. It is healthy. It helps our bodies look beautiful and if these aren't reasons enough . . . *it helps to give us power and control over our lives.*

exercise architecture: building the house of you

· how muscles work ·

brief look into muscle physiology will help you understand how your muscles work and grow.

Your muscles are made up of thousands of individual muscle fibers. Muscle fibers are held together with a complex of connective tissues that fuse together and become tendons at each end of a muscle. Tendons connect your skeletal muscle to your bones. Your limbs move when your tendons change length.

Your muscles will grow when they are challenged—for instance, by participating in a training program featuring dumbbells. The resistance of dumbbells stresses your muscles, creating micro-tears in the fibers. As the muscle fibers heal, three physiologic responses take place:

- Growth
- Revascularization (increased blood flow)
- More efficient use of oxygen

The end product of this muscle reformation is an increase in functional strength. And, not incidentally, all that muscle burns calories like gangbusters.

· building the house of you ·

Your exercise architecture is based on five constructs:

- genetics
- gender
- exercise programming
- exercise design and structure
- your emotional blueprint

GENETICS

"The apple doesn't fall far from the tree." Not original but apropos. The apple may roll off to one side or another. Or even tumble down the hill into an orange grove. It may mingle with other tree fruits or become involved with an avocado. But its shape and color and size and taste are all apple.

The same is true of you. You have a set of predetermined physiologic values. Your stature, bone structure, coloring, body type, and some metabolic characteristics are genetically programmed. You cannot ignore them or change them beyond a certain point. I have tried and tried to stretch my little frame to reach five feet one. But it's not happening. What I have been able to do, though, is build muscle mass, maintain a lean weight, stay functionally fit, keep a relatively flat abdomen for a woman who has had two children, and—this is a big one for me—curtail certain genetically predisposed metabolic problems. My family has a history of hypertension (high blood pressure) and of heart disease. I know this and do everything in my power to protect myself.

What you can do for yourself is work to your genetic potential. In other words, *be the best you can be* (also not an original thought, but one that truly fits). Take control. Be in charge. The genetic-opportunity door swings both ways. There are some people who are genetically gifted and who toss that gift away. And there are some people who are genetically limited and work to full capacity to reap the beautiful benefits.

GENDER

Muscle loves testosterone. It is the hormone most responsible for predicting muscle growth and physical strength. Men have lots of it. Women have a little bit. That is why men are stronger than women. (We're talking physically here. In other arenas, well, that's another book.) The good news is you have enough of this muscle-building hormone to use to your advantage but not enough to become musclebound, a look most women do not want. What we do want are beautiful, lean muscles that make us look sexy and healthy, keep us functionally strong, and help us burn calories.

EXERCISE PROGRAMMING

What you do, how you do it, and how long and how often determine the results you can expect to achieve. Now, this does not mean more is better. Sometimes less is better, if you are training properly and with integrity and, of course, commitment.

There is something called "training specificity." What that means is if you want to run a marathon, you'd better practice running long distances in single bouts. If you want to be a strong recreational tennis player, it won't do your tennis game much good if you practice your golf swing. In other words, and there's no hidden logic here, your body and your neuromuscular system adapt to the appropriate repetitive stimuli.

In order to grow calorie-burning muscle, your dumbbell program should:

- Allow you to build muscle safely and confidently
- Be customized to accomplish your fitness goals
- Take into consideration any areas of injury or weakness
- Be versatile and progressive
- *Be enjoyable!*

EXERCISE DESIGN AND STRUCTURE

A well-designed exercise program is like a well-designed pair of shoes . . . it fits properly, doesn't hurt, gets you where you're going, and makes you look and feel beautiful.

As I will discuss in chapter 3, setting realistic goals is the number one motivational force that will keep you caught up in the cycle of positive momentum I call the Exercise Success Triad. Your goals are your blueprint. And I can't say this enough: To build a proper foundation of health and fitness, your goals must be *realistic*. You wouldn't go out and run a marathon if you'd never even walked a mile.

To help you plot your goals, I ask you to take some time right now to complete the 6-Site Body Evaluation Log at the beginning of the appendix. The only tools required are a tape measure and a scale. And one other thing is required as well: brutal honesty. This is the time to give yourself a serious body evaluation. The best way to take the measurements is sans clothing (that would be naked). But if that feels uncomfortable for you, wear a bathing suit, underwear, or easy-fitting clothes so you can take accurate measurements. Sometimes it is a bit cumbersome to take your own body measurements, holding the tape, wrapping it around you, and trying to read the numbers. If you find it difficult, ask a trusted friend to help you.

After you've done this, take some time for quiet reflection and contemplation. You've got the numbers in front of you. You've got your reality and objectives on paper. The 6-Site Body Evaluation Log is a serious working blueprint. Just like any well thought out architectural plan, it will help you design a program to meet your requirements and fulfill your health-fitness goals. You're building the House of You. Your goal is to build a strong, functional, beautiful body, to live in it with pride and for a long time.

A cautionary word: Do not use the results of these measurements to be hard on yourself or put yourself down. Don't compare yourself to your sister, best friend, or coworker. Women tend to do that—and it's not okay. Everyone—yes, everyone, including celebrities and models we think have bodies as perfect as human bodies have a right to be—finds physical flaws.

Smart Girls take pride in themselves. They take command. They do whatever is necessary to protect their health, their bodies, and their happiness. Smart Girls are their own best friends.

Form and Technique, Form and Technique, Form and Technique

I guess I've made my point. Nothing matters quite as much as learning proper form and technique. Some of the undesirable conscquences of sloppy form and technique are these:

- Increased risk of injury
- Lack of results
- Undesirable results
- Increased stress on low back and joints
- Shortening of full range of motion in joints

Among the benefits of proper form and technique are the following:

- Greater results in a shorter period of time
- Increases in all-over body strengthening
- Less risk of injuring back, neck, spine, hips, and wrists
- Enhanced body awareness and image
- Entrance into the Exercise Success Triad

YOUR EMOTIONAL BLUEPRINT

When I want to achieve some important change in my life, something very meaningful and profound, one of the most powerful tools I use is my journal. Maintaining a diary, journal, log, notebook, exercise bible, whatever you want to call it, serves as both inspiration and consolation.

It will be your personal documentary of a life-altering event. I know we're just dealing with dumbbells here, but I believe, and I hope you're starting to trust me on this, using dumbbells *can* and *will* change not only your body, but also your life.

So I'm going to give you an exercise journal table of contents to help you with basic structure.

You're probably saying, "Hey, Judith, you expect me to do my dumbbell exercises and keep a journal as well? That's asking a lot. Where will I find the time?"

I'm not suggesting you write a dissertation every day in your exercise journal. I'm just suggesting you take a moment, maybe right at the end of your workout, to record your feelings and thoughts. It could be one line: "Today was the first time I saw muscles in the front of my arm!" or "Wow, I increased my weights today. I never thought I'd be able to lift six-pound weights!"

Or, on a day you have extra time, you can be more thorough. There are no rules. And you don't have to write every day. This should be an experience that brings you comfort, emotional support, and continued encouragement.

One of the primary purposes of your Smart Girls exercise journal is to help you keep all your important information together. It will help you chart your progress and witness your success. Think of it as your training partner. Like any good training partner, it will help you stay focused and on track.

I'm going to give you some suggestions and ideas, but primarily this is your creation and inspiration. Remember, this is for *you* and about *you*. It's personal and private, just like any journal or diary. What's inside is no one else's business

I spend a great deal of time pondering the selection of my journal. Just the purchase of it, for me, is a very big deal because I feel I am taking the first step toward a new horizon. Color, size, texture, design, I think about all these things, because I know I am creating a history, not only of my growing strength, but of my emotional well-being. Because you will use your journal frequently, you'll want it to be something special that you enjoy looking at, holding, writing in, and rereading (as time goes on).

How you organize your exercise journal is up to you, but I suggest dividing it into sections. It keeps the information clear and easy to access. I usually have six sections in mine:

1. Personal mission statement
2. Assignments
3. Exercises
4. Exercise schedule
5. Daily workout program
6. Feelings, inspirations, and thoughts (FIT)

1. Personal Mission Statement

Please do not get all worked up over this. It is a brief declaration of desire. It is not a composition about your life's purpose. You can say something simple, like, "I want to look leaner and build muscle because I will look better and be healthier."

The one thing I ask is that you make your personal mission statement positive. No negative personal comments like, "I'm fat and hate my body." That is not a mission statement. Instead, write something positive and inspirational, such as, "I am going to give myself the gift of physical strength and personal power. I deserve it."

No self-indictments! Even though I said this is your journal in which to write anything you want, I do have one rule: You cannot be cruel to yourself. Remember, the mere fact that you are now seriously preparing to embark on an exercise program is an amazing act of self-affirmation.

I gave this journal-writing assignment once to a client by the name of Beth. She got all nervous and upset because she didn't know what she should write. I told her there is no "should."

"Write what you feel and what you want to achieve," I encouraged her. Beth was about thirty-five and was gaining weight and losing muscle and feeling down on herself and, of course, frustrated. "I hardly eat and yet I can't seem to lose weight" (sound familiar?). After doing a body composition test on her, I informed her that her problem was reduced muscle. In order to lose weight, she needed to gain muscle.

When she came to the gym for her next workout, she handed me her personal mission statement. It read: "I don't want to be fat anymore. Also, I want smaller hips and not such a big ass. I'd like to be a size 4 in a couple of weeks."

"Okay, Beth," I said, "this is a great start but it needs to be a bit more positive, more inspirational, more *realistic*." I don't usually do this, but I said, "Let's think about this together."

First I asked her, "What do you like about your body?" Her immediate response was, "Nothing." After we talked a bit, she admitted she had nice arms (which she did). Then we started to redraft her mission statement to embrace a more positive viewpoint. Here is what Beth's mission statement ended up stating: "I have some attractive features and I want to create a more balanced and healthful body."

Now, that is a beautiful personal mission statement.

2. Assignments

This section of your exercise journal includes copies of all the assignments from this book:

- The "I Can't" Grid
- Your 6-Site Body Evaluation Log

From time to time you will want to, and should, monitor your progress. Keeping all your records in one section will make this easier. *Smart Girls* is specifically designed to serve as your "personal trainer" to use in your home gym or take with you to your fitness club or on the road. But still it is a good idea to keep a separate notebook for additional charts and other personal information.

I suggest making copies of all the forms I give you in this book and writing your statistics on the copies. (This way, you can re-create the forms as you need them for documentation.) After three months, your body measurements will probably have changed, so you'll want to keep ongoing records of your changes and progress.

3. Exercises

I have described 30 Smart Girl Dumbbell Exercise Recipes, an additional 5 Dumbbell-Free Exercises, 6 Ab-Flattener Exercise Recipes and 7 All-Purpose Stretch Exercise Recipes. Some of them will feel right for you and some of them won't. I'm going to give you several options for each body part so you'll be able to choose exercises you like to do. You can copy the instructions and illustrations of the exercises you like and place them in your journal. Also, you might want to collect some other exercise ideas from magazines or other books or exercise classes. The more variations you have to select from, the more fun you will have and the easier it will be to adhere to your exercise program. Because—and this is a universal response—boredom is one of the great killers of exercise incentive.

I remember when my children were toddlers someone gave me some excellent advice. "Children grow bored playing with the same toys over and over again, even their favorites. So put them away for a while, hide them out of reach," the day-care director told me. "Then one rainy day when they're cranky and bored playing with the current batch of toys, bring out an old one. It's almost like a new toy all over again, or even better, because they have a pleasant memory of how much they loved the toy when it was brand new."

The same is true of exercises. Some dumbbell exercises you will love doing, and you'll do them over and over again as you see the results start to emerge. But eventually you may tire of them and need a new challenge. So the more variations you have in your exercise arsenal, the easier it is to keep your program fresh, fun, and exciting.

Your exercise journal is the perfect place to save your exercise recipes. Eventually you will have a great and versatile collection that will be an invaluable resource to you.

4. Exercise Schedule

I begin my week by scanning my calendar to see what time each day I'm going to exercise. (Note that I don't look to see *if* I can exercise that day, but what *time* I will be exercising. It's a given on my to do list.) Then I decide on my workout time and block out the time in my calendar, just like any other appointment: business, doctor, hair, family obligation, lunch date.

Your Smart Girls workout program is specifically designed to take you 30 minutes (or less). So, you should be able to fit it in easily sometime during your day on most days of the week. It doesn't matter what time you do it: before work, after school, middle of the day. Your body doesn't care. It only cares that you do it!

The important thing is to be flexible. My preference is to exercise early in the morning on most days. But if I can't, I find the next best time to fit it in. Maybe my session won't be as long, but still, something is better than nothing. (And speaking of "something is better than nothing," that is a mantra I want you to write down somewhere or memorize right now. Here's why: It allows you to embrace whatever exercises you can do that day and, furthermore, it is true.)

Here's what can happen if you're inflexible: Say, for example, you won't work out any time except in the morning (or evening or afternoon). If something happens to prevent you from using that time slot, you then feel you can't exercise at all that day.

Also, on especially busy days, when your schedule becomes overcrowded and you think you have absolutely no time to work out, you *do*. Just pick one or two body parts and work on those. *You don't need to do your entire routine.* Do some biceps curls, some abdominals, and some stretching, and if that's all you can fit in, *good enough!*

The trick to staying in the Exercise Success Triad, is to do what you can each day. I call it your "Cumulative Exercise Output" (CEO). And, as it is for any good CEO running a corporation, it's not just about one day's work or a single effort. It's about the big picture, your long-term success in building and maintaining a life of health, fitness, and self-care.

5. Daily Workout Program

This section of your exercise journal is where you keep a history of your dumbbell workout routines. In the appendix you will find a form, the Daily Dumbbell Workout Schedule, to help you keep accurate records of your exercise program. From day to day, you will record the muscle group you worked, what exercises you did, which weights you used, and how many reps and sets you did.

In addition to the nuts and bolts of your dumbbell workout, I've also included a section for you to record your feelings. I call this the Feelings of Energy Expended. It is a monitoring system to help you evaluate your performance. Here's how it works: After you've completed your dumbbell set, take a moment to reflect and assess *how you feel about how you performed your set*. The appendix contains a "Feelings of Energy Expended" Scale to help you make this assessment. Rate the quality of your effort, using a scale of values from 3 to 12. Some days you may give yourself a rating of 3 or 4 and some days you may give yourself a rating of 10 or 12.

Again, it is important not to use this energy-monitoring device to be hard on yourself about your workout. It is a feedback mechanism to help you honestly evaluate and enhance your performance. My own coach once said to me during the last reps on my last set when I was starting to lose energy and form, "You're doing them anyway so make each rep count."

You might be asking yourself why the scale starts at 3 and not 1. I think the mere fact that you've taken the time to use your dumbbells, that you've gone into your workout area and picked them up, deserves a huge amount of credit. Because the truth is, it is harder to get going than to keep going.

6. Feelings, Inspirations, and Thoughts (FIT)

This section of your exercise journal has nothing to do with exercise. But it has a lot to do with your spiritual self, which I think is equally important; and, of course, with the intimate and profound connection between your body and your mind.

What is the connection between physical strength and spiritual well-being? Our spirit is our essence. It is our internal guardian. It is the animating principle infusing our physical being. If your physical being is weak or vulnerable, if it causes you shame or fails to allow you to participate in the world in a powerful way, your sense of well-being suffers. Protecting your health, building strength, feeling physically in control are direct responses to exercise. A strong physical being is the structure in which a sound spirit resides and soars.

In his book *The 7 Habits of Highly Effective People*, Stephen Covey calls it "sharpening the saw." He asks: How is it possible to be an effective human being if we are working with ineffective equipment?

This is a place in your journal to collect thoughts, words, or images—anything that motivates or touches you spiritually or emotionally. (For instance, I keep the Covey quote in my journal.) It might be a favorite photograph of yourself or a quote from Emerson or Plato or lyrics from Sting. Perhaps something a friend or teacher, poet, or colleague said that made sense. We are each emotionally touched or spiritually moved in our own way. For example, I love words. Since I was a teenager, I collected word journals. If I heard a word or read a sentence or a quote that I thought was powerful or beautiful, or that lucidly expressed some emotion I myself was unable to express, I wrote it down in a little black notebook.

This is also the place to write down your thoughts and feelings about your experience as you start to change your life and become healthier. Maybe *Smart Girls Do Dumbbells* is the first fitness book you've ever bought, or maybe this is what feels like the hundredth time you've tried to stay committed to an exercise program. Write down your feelings about this: your expectations, frustrations, aspirations, feelings of success, feelings of failure, feelings about anything you have feelings about. It doesn't have to be just about your exercise.

In the next chapter, I am going to unveil the key elements of exercise success in the Exercise Success Triad. Once you begin to fully understand why it was hard for you to keep up with your exercise programs in the past, and how you can master the art and discipline of exercise in the future, you will be on your way to the lifelong practice of fitness and strength.

the exercise success triad

have found, from the patients I work with at UCLA and the nearly two decades I have been in private practice, that long-term exercisers have become so because of three contiguous elements: knowledge, results, and consistency. I call this the Exercise Success Triad.

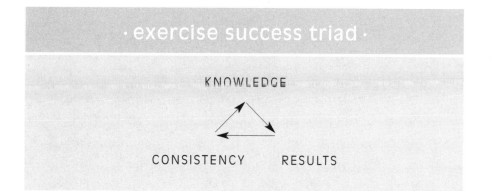

· exercise success triad ·

KNOWLEDGE

CONSISTENCY   RESULTS

These three elements are on a continuum, affecting your exercise success in the following way: *Knowledge,* understanding how to do exercise correctly, creates *results,* which leads to *consistency,* which spurs a desire for increased knowledge, and so forth.

· the exercise success triad: knowledge ·

There are two ways to learn a skill, or learn anything for that matter: the correct way and the incorrect way. Sometimes learning something the wrong way is not critical. For instance, applying eyeliner—I always have trouble getting that thin little line close to my lashes. So, the worst that happens because of my lack of skill is that sometimes I look like a clown. But sometimes lack of knowledge can be counterproductive, not to mention dangerous. Learning exercise form and technique properly is important for two reasons: It ensures results and prevents injury.

I give you detailed instructions on proper form and technique in chapter 10 on the Smart Girls dumbbell exercise recipes. Once you've mastered these skills, they are lifelong abilities. *Knowledge* is the first, most critical step because it will lead you directly to *Results*.

· the exercise success triad: results ·

We all function on an effort-reward continuum. If I do certain actions, I expect certain results. If I study the course material hard enough, I will pass the test. If I follow the recipe properly, the soufflé won't collapse. If I take the time and effort to exercise, I will lose weight and improve my health. Makes sense, yes? But what if you studied only half the material or the wrong material? Or you didn't beat the egg whites long enough? And what if you took the time to exercise religiously, overcoming your own prejudices about how you dislike it, forcing yourself to get up a bit earlier or stay up a little later, and three months down the exercise road you looked the same as you did when you started? You'd say, "Well, this isn't working," and give up. I wouldn't blame you. You'd be working on a frustrating paradigm: maximum effort = minimum reward

The Exercise Success Triad is an interactive paradigm. If you lift the dumbbells properly, you will achieve results. Once you've seen results, you will be loath to relinquish them. Then you are inspired to stick with them consistently. Greater consistency leads to a quest for more knowledge, which generates more results.

· the exercise success triad: consistency ·

Consistency is a direct by-product of results. "Ah, this is working. I think I'll keep doing it!"

In my gym, consistency is king. I don't care if one of my clients misses a session or even a couple of sessions. Taking a little hiatus, a week or two, from exercise is okay. Taking a permanent vacation is not.

I am often asked how I exercise every day. Here's what I have discovered, and I think you'll understand: It is easier to *continue* exercising, even if it's doing just a little something each day, than to stop and start again. When you think about this you know it is true. What's one of the hardest things in the world to do? Go back to work after a long holiday. It doesn't even have to be a long holiday. Monday mornings are notoriously ugly days because you've had two days of freedom and relaxation. I'm not saying give up your weekends or holidays to work, but I'll leave you with a quote from Horace: "Once begun, a task is easy; half the work is done."

Dr. David Heber, director of the UCLA Center for Human Nutrition and an expert in weight loss and nutrition, says, "Exercise is the only healthy addiction." The question is: How does one become addicted?

One way to become "addicted" is to activate what I call "motivational forces." These are sort of inspiration cues, methods to keep you going even during those commitment doldrums. There are ten Motivational Forces that serve as invaluable little behavioral links, like stepping-stones, that keep you hooked on exercise and on the path to consistency.

10 SMART GIRL MOTIVATIONAL FORCES

1. Set realistic goals
2. Readjust your concept of exercise
3. Delete guilt
4. Be flexible, think creatively
5. Go for convenience
6. Practice patience
7. Think the big picture—CEO
8. Take pride
9. Don't give up
10. Enjoy the high

SET REALISTIC GOALS

I am petite: 60 inches. 1.5 meters. 152.5 centimeters. Five feet *nothing*. That's all there is. Sometimes I lie and say I'm five feet and a half—that's usually around someone who is spatially impaired or not carrying a tape measure. I must confess there are times I wish I were a little taller, especially when I see a very attractive six-foot man. There's another reason, as well, a more serious and important one. Height loss is one of the serious consequences of the aging process. When one tops out at five feet, one can't afford to lose even a centimeter of height. So, even though I do a lot of stretching and protect my spine and bones by doing my dumbbell exercises, practicing good posture, and getting sufficient calcium, I'm not doing these things because they will help me get taller. That's an unrealistic expectation. I'm doing them to help prevent me from getting *smaller!*

Nellie came to see me because she was unhappy about her weight. She is five feet six inches tall and thirty-four years old. "I want to weigh 105 pounds," she told me. "Have you ever weighed 105 pounds?" I asked.

"No, but I once weighed 110. I was right out of college when I first started working. Then I got married, had the kids, you know." She did need to lose weight, but it was very unlikely Nellie was going to weigh 105 pounds. It was an unrealistic goal. In order for her to be successful with her weight loss and exercise program, she had to set a realistic goal.

The consequence of setting unrealistic fitness goals is the antithesis of being in the Exercise Success Triad. I call it the Exercise Failure Syndrome.

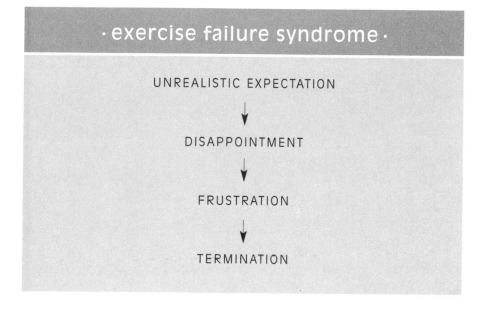

How do you set realistic goals? You examine your 6-Site Body Evaluation Log carefully. You have an honest talk with yourself. Following are some of the questions you should be asking:

- Am I trying to alter a genetic trait?
- Is this something I can do without hurting myself, physically or emotionally?
- Can I make this a part of a permanent lifestyle change?
- Am I hung up on numbers or will I be satisfied with a course of exercise that improves my health, my body, my sense of self-worth, and my personal power?

READJUST YOUR CONCEPT OF EXERCISE

Here's a bit of good news I think you're really going to enjoy hearing: Your workout doesn't always have to take a lot of time and it doesn't have to be painful or boring. It doesn't require an expensive gym membership or fancy equipment. It requires only a serious commitment to a well-designed workout program and the willingness to reap the benefits.

What it does take is *integrity*. Each time you lift your dumbbells make every rep count . . . even if you're only doing it for fifteen minutes.

For cardiovascular fitness—walking, jogging, swimming, biking—the American College of Sports Medicine prescribes the following:

FREQUENCY: All or most days of the week

INTENSITY: 60 to 90 percent of maximal heart rate

DURATION: 15 to 60 minutes

MODE: Using large muscle groups in rhythmic motion

Your maximal heart rate (MHR) is age predicted. The formula to calibrate your MHR is:

220 minus your age.

Example: You are thirty years old. Your MHR is 190.

Exercising to your MHR is usually done in a clinical setting to test the heart muscle. Fitness exercisers use only a percentage of the MHR. Using the example above, if you are thirty years old and wanted to use 70 percent of your MHR you would multiply 190 by .70, which would be 133 beats per minute.

Pick an aerobic activity that you enjoy. Don't discount any physical activity because it doesn't fit your image of yourself or what you have been told exercise "should be."

"I don't do any exercise," Jill told me. I was sort of surprised because she looked healthy and had a great shape, and I was wondering how she got that way doing *nothing*.

"Well, you look great" was my honest appraisal. "So you don't do any recreational activities?" I asked.

"Oh, I square-dance three or four times a week."

"What! You told me you didn't do any exercise."

"That's not exercise, that's square dancing. It's fun."

"But it *is* exercise! It is aerobic exercise absolutely!"

Jill's square dancing meets all the criteria. She is using large muscle groups (her legs) consistently in a rhythmic fashion for a steady period of time.

She was surprised to find she was already into the Exercise Success Triad. And I explained that building muscles using dumbbells was actually going to help her with square dancing. "It will allow you to keep your leg muscles strong and the connective tissues around your joints fluid and flexible. You'll be square dancing for a long time."

With this, she was ready to begin working with the dumbbells.

DELETE GUILT

Most everyone feels guilty about their exercise, or lack thereof. (Even I do occasionally.) You think you're not doing it long enough or right enough or hard enough.

"I only did my weights for fifteen minutes the other day," Carla tells me. "I know that wasn't enough."

"Did you make each rep count? Concentrate and work with good form and technique? Maintain good posture and use correct breathing?"

"Yeah, but I ran out of time and I felt guilty about not doing my whole set."

"Here's when you're allowed to feel guilty," I told her. "If instead of using those fifteen minutes to do part of your workout, you decide instead to sit down and watch the shopping network, or order food online, then you have permission to feel guilty."

Guilt is self-defeating and counterproductive. And it can lead you into the Exercise Failure Syndrome because you become frustrated, which, as you know, leads to disappointment, which leads to termination.

Instead, if you have a time crunch, *do the best you can in the time you have.*

That's it. Don't drag around negative feelings and a sense of failure. Instead, congratulate yourself for using minimum time for maximum benefits. You did something wonderful for yourself and your body with the time you had. Congratulations!

BE FLEXIBLE, THINK CREATIVELY

Here are the two complaints I hear most: "Exercise is boring" and "I'm tired of chicken." (The latter one is from my teenage son when I tell him what I'm preparing for dinner.)

At any rate, I have already agreed exercise can be boring. What makes it boring is doing the same exercises over and over and over again, year after year after year. No surprises here. You wouldn't watch the same film or read the same novel or eat the same meal over and over again, would you? So, if you're bored with your workout . . . *change it!*

The problem is, all of us tend to stay within our comfort zones. We stick with what is familiar because, well, it *is* familiar, it's safe. We're afraid to venture out, to try new modes of exercise because we are afraid of looking silly, being clumsy, feeling uncomfortable. Or worse, we're just too lazy to try something new.

One way to avoid exercise boredom syndrome is to think of creative new ways to exercise. In this book you are going to learn thirty Dumbbell Exercise Recipes, five Dumbbell-Free Exercise Recipes, six Ab-Flattening Exercise Recipes, and seven All-Purpose Stretch Recipes to keep your program fresh and interesting. If you're bored doing biceps curls one way then do them another. Experiment. Have fun. Be flexible. Add in a new exercise or rearrange the order. New forms of exercise stimulate muscles and target them in new ways, increasing your skill level and enhancing results.

If you try a new form of exercise and you don't like it, don't do it again. Never force yourself to do any exercise that hurts or doesn't suit your needs. You will discover there are many different dumbbell exercises that will accomplish your goals. Try them out. See which feel right. Ask yourself if you're getting the results you want. Be flexible, think creatively!

GO FOR CONVENIENCE

I say if you have to travel more than fifteen minutes to get to your workout, you probably won't get there. Not on a regular basis, as part of your life, that is. None of us has time to spare. If your workout time is increased by commute time, it's not going to work for you in the long run. The whole idea here is to fit exercise into your life on a *consistent* basis as *conveniently* as possible.

If you are going to do your workout at a commercial gym, join one as close to home as possible. If there isn't a facility close by, join one close to work. Also, look into your local YMCA. To find the nearest YMCA, call 1-888-333-YMCA or log on to www.YMCA.net.

You can also work out right in your own home with no travel time, no membership fee, no prying eyes. If you want to create a home gym, you will be most interested in chapter 9 "Building Your Personalized Dumbbell Gym." I think you'll be in for some nice surprises, too. It's not going to cost you a lot of money, less than a hundred dollars. You don't need elaborate equipment that takes up a lot of space. It can all be done in a small corner of any room: den, dorm, office, bedroom.

PRACTICE PATIENCE

"So how long before this flab disappears from the backs of my arms?" Lily asks me. We were at a party at the time drinking wine coolers and eating guacamole and chips. "Well, first it might be a good idea for you to visit me in the gym so we can get started."

When people find out what I do I spend a lot of my off-hours answering questions just like Lily's.

They always remind me of the joke about the woman who wanted to win the lottery and prayed to God week after week to answer her prayers and help her win. Finally God got really frustrated with her and said, "Could you help me out here and at least buy a ticket?"

As I have said, there are no instant results. There are no easy answers.

There are no get-fit-quick gimmicks that are really going to give you the results you want long-term.

That said, let me give you a few facts about muscle physiology. When you start an exercise regimen, the first adaptations are neuromuscular. That means your body's central nervous system starts to adapt to new stimuli. So even if there's no visual evidence of all your efforts, changes *are* happening. Very important ones. You will start to see visual changes—less flab, more muscle delineation (cuts), and hypertrophy (muscle growth)—in about twelve to sixteen weeks, that is, if you are *consistent* and *committed*.

Results are a *reality*.

THINK THE BIG PICTURE—CEO

"I can't see you for the next couple of weeks," Anna tells me. "My manager quit and I have to be at the store and look for a new manager. The holidays are coming. I don't have a spare moment for anything but work and the kids. Exercise is not going to happen," she said.

She had made incredible progress in the last three months and I could tell she was distraught about stopping. So, instead of going through her regular workout, we spent that session modifying her program to fit into her life for the next few weeks so she didn't have to stop exercising entirely. It's sort of like elite athletes off-season. They don't train as much or as hard as when they're competing, but they do a modified workout to remain fit, strong, and flexible so it's not so difficult to get back into shape when they return to training camp. Athletic trainers call it "periodization." I call it Cumulative Exercise Output (CEO). CEO allows you to rethink the meaning of exercise because it is not about a single bout or one week or one month. It's about allowing yourself to be flexible so exercise fits into your life long-term. It is not about the moment; it's about a permanent lifestyle change.

Not enough time to work out? Fine! I have given you special selections of exercise recipes in your 30-Day menu to get you through those times. There is Something Is Better than Nothing Day, Tide Me Over Day, and A Little Goes a Long Way Day. These are sort of "exercise quickies" to get you through time-challenged or low-energy days and keep you in the Exercise Success Triad.

I think this quote about the value of possessing a flexible mind-set, from Charles F. Kettering in *Profile of America,* sums it up: "Where there is an open mind, there will always be a frontier."

Thinking CEO gives you the liberty of viewing your exercise habit with an open mind in a flexible way. You're not hard on yourself if you miss a session because you know you'll make up for it later. I find most people are extremely hard on themselves when it comes to exercise. This is especially true of women. We think we're not doing it well enough or hard enough or long enough, so we end up giving up altogether. Which leads me to the next motivational force: healthy pride.

TAKE PRIDE

There are no small accomplishments, only small attitudes. Each time you manage to lift those dumbbells, take a walk, or go to the gym, own that accomplishment. If you usually walk for thirty minutes a day and on a certain day you can only walk for fifteen or twenty minutes, congratulate yourself on making the effort. If one week you make it to the gym five times and the next you only make it twice—and you've been honest about your effort—then you've done the best you can for that week and that *is good enough.* Each time you fulfill your commitment to yourself it is important to own that accomplishment, trust you're doing the best you can do, and take pride in yourself.

Each day, you are faced with new decisions and demands on your time. Each day you have a choice whether you are going to do something healthy and healing for yourself or neglect yourself.

DON'T GIVE UP

We all have down times. Trust yourself. Believe that you are doing the best you can during your down times, because you are. You only have one person to answer to: you. Becoming strong and fit and healthy is not just about reaching a goal. It is about pursuing a lifestyle.

Nineteenth-century poet and essayist Leigh Hunt wrote, "Patience and gentleness is power." Be patient. Be gentle. These traits, combined with your commitment to your health, are some of the greatest gifts you can bestow upon yourself.

ENJOY THE HIGH

Clinical trials as well as observational studies show that physical activity helps reduce stress levels. It has also been shown to lessen symptoms of depression. An article that appeared in *Medicine and Science in Sports and Exercise,* on the impact of physical activity and depression, concluded that "light, moderate, and vigorous intensity exercise can reduce symptoms of depression."

As a physiological response to endurance activities, a part of our brain, the hypothalamus, releases hormones called endorphins or beta endorphins that make us feel better and more serene. It makes sense—a walk around the block is a whole lot healthier than a walk to the medicine chest. Additionally, you're not only increasing feelings of well-being and reducing your stress level, you're burning calories, working your heart, and using your lungs.

If you go for a walk or a jog, or do your dumbbell exercises, I guarantee that when you are finished, you will feel better physically and emotionally. Exercise is a great way to clear your head, stimulate ideas, and solve problems. I am not suggesting that lifting your dumbbells can lift all stressful situations. But working out is an excellent antianxiety, antidepressant activity.

How does exercise help battle depression? In a study published in the *British Journal of Sports Medicine,* it was suggested that a natural stimulant produced by the body, phenylethylamine (PEA), increases through moderate exercise. The researchers concluded that "the antidepressant effects of exercise appear to be linked to increased phenylethylamine concentrations." These increases may be responsible for feelings of "euphoria," often called "runner's high." People suffering from depression tend to have low PEA levels. That may explain why exercise has been credited with serving as a *natural* antidepressant. PEA increases may be the reward we give ourselves for exercising! So if after your workout you think you're feeling better physically, mentally, and emotionally, you are. Enjoy!

· all days are not created equal ·

Your energy level, skill, and strength shift from day to day. This is as true for highly trained athletes as for the general population participating in health-fitness programs. One day your favorite ballplayer is a bum, and the next he's a hero. Give yourself a break. If your energy level is a little low, or your schedule doesn't permit you to do your full workout, or if you're simply overwhelmed by life, as we all are from time to time . . . do what you can.

You also may experience some interesting surprises. You may have a most unexpected energy surge. For instance, upon your return to your exercise program following a break, you might think, "Oh, I'm not going to have much strength, I haven't trained in a week." But you might be pleasantly surprised to find you haven't lost any strength, but may have even more power—and a renewed enthusiasm—than before your hiatus.

And then there are stressful days. Your computer crashes or, worse, it doesn't crash so you have no excuse not to finish the report that is currently ten days past due. Days when your mental energy output has been so extreme that you think you'll have little physical strength remaining. You drag yourself over to your dumbbells and, wow . . . not only are you pumping well, you've sort of forgotten the annoyances of the day. What a great transformation!

Motivation requires an intrinsic belief that exercise is important and a willingness to incorporate changes in your life for your health. When I lecture I ask, "How many of you believe exercise is important?" One hundred percent of my audience raise their hands. When I ask, "How many of you are currently exercising on a regular basis?" sadly my yield drops to about 40 percent.

When it comes to exercise there is what I call an "execution gap." Not a lack of understanding, but a lack of implementation. Why? And how are you going to bridge that gap?

· 4 ·

you
are your own
best coach

exercise sucks. Not all the time. But sometimes it sure does. Also, you think it's boring. Well, yeah, it can be boring. It isn't always easy or fun. Results don't happen overnight. And once you've reached your goals, you're still not done. You have to keep on lifting those dumbbells, or the beautiful gains will slowly vanish.

There are some lies, too. I'm telling you right now: Don't believe get-fit-quick articles. It doesn't happen that way. Don't believe books that offer fast remedies or exercise made easy. Muscle-zapping electrodes that move your muscles for you while you sip a glass of Chardonnay and recline in front of the TV, and supplements that claim to build muscle while you sleep. Trash. There's no way around it: Exercise is, well, *exercise*. And it is eternal—a permanent lifestyle intervention that will change your body, your health, your life, and even your disposition . . . *but it only works as long as you do the work.*

That said, some days you're really going to love it, I promise. And you're going to love the way you look and feel, *guaranteed!* Your body will be leaner, your clothes will fit better, your energy level will be higher, your attitude more positive. You're going to walk away from those dumbbells with an amazing sense of accomplishment. Your body will be stronger. But that's not all. You will feel a sense of personal power. It is the highest high you can imagine: personal physical and emotional strength.

· sure it's hard, but it really does come naturally ·

Our bodies are designed to move. That's what muscles are made for. And I have found most people learn how to exercise quickly. There are important reminders about form and technique that consistently need reinforcing, but our bodies move naturally. Past a certain age, we all know how to flex and extend our hips to walk. We know how to flex our shoulder and extend our elbow so we can blow-dry our hair, and we know how to extend our knee to admire a new pair of shoes. These movements are automatic reflexes of our central nervous system. You don't think about them, you just do them.

Exercise is a formal, more concentrated version of our natural body movements. For instance, if you want to get rid of that nasty flab hanging off the undersides of your arms, you extend your elbow while adding some resistance, dumbbells, for example. You can also use your own body weight as resistance simply by doing push-ups.

If we all know how to move, and we all need to move in order to accomplish everyday tasks, from eating to writing to playing tennis, what's the problem? Why is this "exercise" business so daunting?

· the "i can't" chant ·

It drums in your head . . . the negative *tumtumtum* . . . I can't, I can't, I can't. Hear it? That niggling little voice perpetuating your self-designated failures and worst disappointments. "I can't . . ." You fill in the rest. The "I Can't" Chant is highly customized, sort of like a finely tailored dress. I can't:

- Find the time to exercise
- Stop smoking
- Start going to the gym
- End a bad relationship
- Start a new relationship
- Save money
- Spend time on myself
- Put down the pie
- Pick up that dumbbell

Few of us are immune to that nasty little voice singing the "I Can't" Chant. It has an all too familiar tone. Whose voice is that, anyway? Precisely who is telling you what you cannot do? Who is holding the baton conducting "I can't, I can't, I can't"? Parents? Husband? Ex-husband? Boyfriend? Lover? Children? Culture?

That voice drumming within our heads is usually our *own*.

It is your choice to allow the voice to chant within you. You can feed into its self-destructive message or you can simply tell it to stop and begin to listen to a new, healthier voice that also resides within you: *I can!*

I can:

- Look better
- Feel better
- Be healthier
- Lift those dumbbells
- Take a walk
- Go for a jog
- Be stronger
- Maintain my resolve

- Not give up
- Not be hard on myself
- Think I'm amazing
- Appreciate my strength
- Value my power
- *Be in charge of me!*

Here's what you want to do right now: Start changing your "I can'ts" into "I cans." The first step is identifying the origin of the "I can'ts." Are they coming from a place of inability? A place of fear? Or maybe from a preconceived notion about what, as a woman, is physically, culturally, or socially acceptable?

Let me tell you Gail's story. She is in her late thirties. She is in good health, but needs to lose about twenty-five pounds. And she's out of condition. "My back hurts when I bend down to pull up my pantyhose. And sometimes it feels like a struggle to lift the grocery bags out of the car. I think the box people pack them too heavy," she said.

I suggested that in addition to a cardiovascular workout she should work on increasing her lean mass.

"You need to start building muscle," I told her.

"You mean weight lifting? Oh, no. I can't. I'm too weak."

"Have you ever lifted dumbbells?"

"I don't even lift a liter of water."

"How do you know you're too weak then?" I ask.

"I just am."

Gail has a thriving career. She is the vice president of a large international advertising firm. She landed the job in an interesting way. She started as an administrative assistant, and one day a junior account executive position opened up on one of the agency's largest accounts, a cosmetics manufacturer. She applied for the job, and in her interview the head of personnel asked why she thought she was qualified for a job for which she had no training, education, or related experience. She replied, "I wear lipstick, don't I? And have you ever noticed, it's a different shade every day?"

When she told me this story of her climb up the corporate ladder, I asked her how she knew she could actually *do* the job. (Frankly, the ability to apply lipstick didn't seem like much of a résumé rouser to me.)

"I didn't. But I thought I didn't have much to lose if I gave it a try. I could always be a secretary again."

"Well, the same is true of lifting dumbbells," I told her. "Give them a try. You don't have much to lose. On the contrary, you have a *lot* to gain. And you can always put them down again."

Gail's "I can't" about lifting weights stemmed from her perception of "not being strong enough." Her thinking is not atypical. A lot of women feel that muscle belongs to men. It's a "men only" club. Wrong. That's a myth we want to dispatch immediately. Muscle is an equal opportunity tissue. It does not *gender* or *age* discriminate. It is ready to work when you are.

I promised Gail and I promise you: As you do the dumbbell exercises in this book, as you feel your body gain strength and power, you will feel a greater sense of power in other aspects of your life, as well. Physical strength gives us both physical and personal power. Power gives us courage. Courage gives us control. Men have always known muscle means power way beyond the physical. There is a huge psychological component. For many women, this is a relatively new concept and one that seems elusive. One of the benefits of our work together is to help build your physical strength and, in doing so, help you access your personal power.

· understanding your own "i can'ts" ·

Before you read any further, I'd like you to make a list on the "I Can't" Grid on page 41. It is important to take some time to think seriously about the "I can'ts" you've programmed into your belief system. It requires total honesty to separate your "I can'ts" from the "I don't feel likes" and the "I don't want tos" and the "I'm just too lazys."

Writing this list offers you a chance to examine more closely what is stopping you from pursuing a healthier lifestyle and to separate myth from reality. Take a moment now to write your list of "I can'ts." Think carefully and *honestly* about the limiting factors you place on yourself—your health, your life, and your attitude.

There is a secret to this exercise business. The magic answer to the magic bullet. I'd like you to keep this secret in mind while reading this book, and long after you put it down. If indeed exercise is the cure, the person in charge of the healing is *you.* That's it . . . there's not a person in the world, no matter how much they care about you or love you, who can make you do it but you. To look at it in a really self-centered way: It's the one area in your life where you can allow yourself to be completely and totally selfish. The time you spend exercising is your gift to yourself. The benefits are so profound, and numerous, anyone who does not take advantage of exercise is saying, "I don't like myself much."

The other very important point is, and I hope you're not going to find this discouraging: It is *never ending,* which sounds worse than it is. It's not a commitment as much as a recommitment, continuous and ongoing. You make it, or more accurately remake it, *every single day.* Because every single day you have to make an exercise appointment with yourself; you have to pull on those running shoes; pick up those dumbbells; push those pedals. You have to drag yourself out of your warm, cozy bed in the morning or drag your tired self to the gym after a long day at school or with the kids or at the office. I've been doing this for almost two decades. Admittedly, it's not always easy, but it is always, *always* worth the effort. I can't think of a time when I have forced myself to work out that I didn't feel better afterward, physically and emotionally.

I heard a great story about what it takes to excel. A world-renowned concert pianist was talking about her early training and how often she practiced. She told the story of her first piano teacher. "I asked him," she said, "how often I would have to practice."

"Only," he replied, "on the days that you eat."

That's the same way I feel about exercise.

Remember, this is for you and about you! No one is judging or evaluating

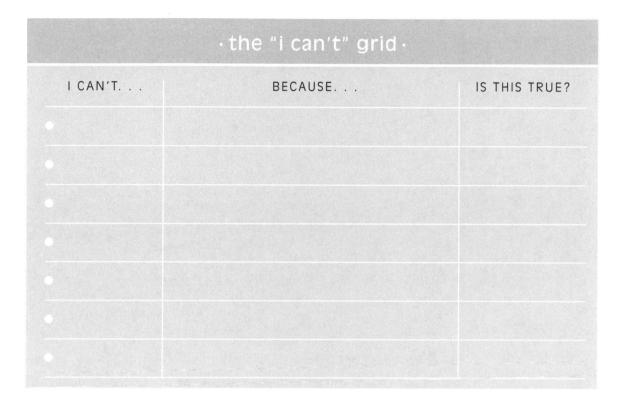

· the "i can't" grid ·		
I CAN'T. . .	BECAUSE. . .	IS THIS TRUE?

you. Once you've completed this list, do not refer to it again for a while. Simply lock it away. Allow yourself time to start gaining your physical strength. Then at some time in the future, decide on the appropriate moment and turn back to this page to examine your list of "I can'ts." I think you'll be surprised at what you find. Some "I can'ts" don't fit any longer. Giving yourself the opportunity to chart your growth is vitally important. It shows you what is possible. And once you've tasted the transformation of *possible* almost nothing seems *impossible*.

· holding on to motivation ·

This is what I hear a lot: "I know I should exercise, but I don't have enough time." This is also very popular: "I know I should exercise, but I don't know how to get motivated." Followed by this famous complaint: "I hate it." (Now you understand what makes my job so difficult. People aren't always thrilled with what I have to offer.)

So the question remains: How do you stay motivated? Maybe even more importantly, how do you even *get* motivated when:

- You don't have a lot of time
- You don't have a lot of tolerance for exercise
- You don't know what you're doing

What is the secret? What is the elusive motivator that allows some people to place those dumbbells in their hands and do those biceps curls day after day, year after year? And how can you get some of it so the task of being healthier, leaner, stronger, and happier doesn't seem so overwhelming?

I've got some good news for you: You are on your way right now! You're reading this book. (And I promise you it has a wonderful ending . . . a healthier, more fabulous you!) You are seeking to make positive changes. The *desire* to change is the most critical first step in the process of change. But you also have to understand some of your inner beliefs.

Our task in the next chapter is to try to understand your personal exercise psychology. You're going to discover right now how you really feel about exercise and your readiness to begin a course of lifelong health and fitness.

how do you feel about exercise?

"Change equals death," director Woody Allen's character remarks in his film *Husbands and Wives*. It might not be *that* drastic, but dealing with change and making changes are significant challenges for most of us. My spiritual mentor once told me, "You won't make any change in your life until you are absolutely ready to do so. It won't happen a minute sooner." "How will I know when that time has come?" I asked. "You won't need to know . . . you'll be doing it."

We all reach moments of personal truth—revelations or clarity about ourselves and what it is that we want. Sometimes the moment comes when we are at an apex of frustration, a point beyond which we are simply no longer willing to tolerate the status quo. And the thing is, no one can tell you when that time is. Not your well-intentioned best friend, your husband, your children, your parents. No one can force you to start the process of change except *you*. And, like my guru said, you will know when that time has come because you'll already be making the changes.

On the next page is a questionnaire on your readiness to begin incorporating the Smart Girls dumbbell workout into your life. Please take the time to consider your answers carefully. Don't judge or evaluate your responses. Simply answer the questions honestly. It will help clarify how you feel about exercise and how emotionally prepared you are to embrace a life-altering exercise regimen in a permanent way.

· exercise readiness questionnaire ·

Compared to previous attempts, how motivated are you this time to begin an exercise program?

1. Not at all
2. Slightly motivated
3. Somewhat motivated
4. Quite motivated
5. Extremely motivated

Are you confident you can fit physical activity into your life regularly?

1. Not at all confident
2. Slightly confident
3. Somewhat confident
4. Highly confident
5. Completely confident

Do you believe exercise is physically painful?

1. Very painful
2. Slightly painful
3. Somewhat painful

4. Not very painful
5. Not painful at all

When you think about exercise, do you develop a positive or negative picture in your mind?

1. Completely negative
2. Somewhat negative
3. Neutral
4. Somewhat positive
5. Completely positive

Are you uncomfortable perspiring while exercising?

1. Very uncomfortable
2. Slightly uncomfortable
3. Somewhat uncomfortable
4. Not very uncomfortable
5. Not at all uncomfortable

Do you believe exercise can be enjoyable?

1. Never
2. Rarely
3. Occasionally
4. Frequently
5. Always

Do you believe exercise is an important factor in weight control and management?

1. Not at all important
2. Slightly important
3. Somewhat important
4. Highly important
5. Vitally important

Do you believe regular exercise is an important factor in maintaining overall health?

1. Not at all important
2. Slightly important
3. Somewhat important
4. Very important
5. Critically important

Do you believe that you can work your Smart Girls dumbbell exercise program into your daily schedule?

1. Not at all certain
2. Slightly certain
3. Somewhat certain
4. Highly certain
5. Completely certain

Do you believe improvements in your health and appearance are realistic outcomes of your Smart Girls dumbbell exercise program?

1. Not at all realistic
2. Slightly realistic
3. Somewhat realistic
4. Highly realistic
5. Completely realistic

EVALUATING YOUR READINESS TO EXERCISE

Total your score by adding together the numbers that you circled in response to each question.

If your score is less than 25: Exercise is challenging for you. Perhaps you have had negative experiences in the past or have been frustrated by the process. The good news is you believe physical activity is necessary to improve and maintain your health, and firm and tone your body. It is important to begin your fitness program very slowly; select only physical activities you enjoy and can tolerate. Be patient with yourself. You are on your way!

If your score is 25 to 40: You have some mixed feelings about exercise but more positive than negative because you understand how important it is. You have a true desire to look and feel better and you know exercise is the answer. Even though you find it challenging sometimes, you are committed to making exercise a permanent part of your life.

If your score is over 40: You enjoy exercise and physical activity. You are probably already participating in a structured program. You enjoy learning new exercise techniques and like being challenged. With your enthusiasm and commitment to health fitness, you would make someone a good training partner.

This should give you some insight into your feelings about exercise. Once you begin to understand your exercise psychology, it should become easier to appreciate your exercise reservations and excuses. Let's face it, if you don't believe exercise is going to make a difference in your health and your life you'll hardly be motivated to lace up your running shoes and head to the track. If you find it painful or are afraid you might feel pain, it will certainly affect your energy and enthusiasm to lift up those dumbbells.

Once you understand your true feelings, there's the opportunity to work with and change your "I can'ts" into "I cans." Perhaps you didn't understand you were coming from a negative psychological place. Maybe you attributed your past lack of success to a genetic weakness or laziness, rather than the truth: that you did not believe a course of fitness and health was really going to make a discernible difference in your life.

If you're prepared and ready to begin, you're going to love the next chapter because you are going to learn why dumbbells are the ideal piece of exercise equipment for Smart Girls to build beautiful muscles.

· 6 ·

why smart girls
do dumbbells

· dumbbells give results! ·

Well, actually, to be more precise, dumbbell exercises. Because the dumbbells themselves, sitting alone unused in the corner of your bedroom or dorm room or office, aren't going to give you muscle. No, you need to pick them up first. This is critical for any sort of success. And, of course, as mentioned earlier, you need to pick them up consistently and with good form and technique if you are going to create the results you desire, and find yourself in the Exercise Success Triad.

Are dumbbells the only resistant mechanism that will help you build muscle? No. There are several different types of resistance mechanisms that load the muscle. But the number one reason to use dumbbells is . . . *results!*

They work. It's that simple. Yes, they are also convenient, inexpensive, and fun. But the primary reason is that *you get results*. They offer many exercise benefits and options in addition to providing you with an excellent workout. I love teaching people how to use dumbbells because once they master form and technique, there is nothing stopping them. They can enhance their workout program at their own speed and comfort level even in their own homes. There is a keen psychological component as well. No matter how many pounds you're lifting (and I have started some women with little one-pounders), you feel an amazing sense of strength. There is a mystique to lifting dumbbells. The mere girth and form of the dumbbells in your hands give you a sense of power.

· dumbbells—also called *free weights*—set you free ·

Remember the White Rabbit in *Alice in Wonderland,* who was holding his timepiece and scurrying about lamenting, "I'm late, I'm late, no time to say hello good-bye, I'm late, I'm late, I'm late?" That's sort of the way a lot of us lead our lives. It feels as if there is never enough time for anything, and yet at day's end, we often ponder, "Why didn't I accomplish what I set out to do today?"

This is one of my favorite nursery rhymes, which I think says it all, for most of us:

> *How pleasant it is at the end of the day,*
> *No follies to have to repent;*
> *But reflect on the past and be able to say,*
> *That my time has been properly spent.*

"Properly spent." Don't you love that? Quality time, this is what this book is about. Perhaps more specifically, *quality exercise time.*

"Love to do it—know I should—would . . . no time." It is the de facto, all-time number one excuse for not exercising. Part of the problem is your concept of what constitutes a proper course of exercise . . . how long, how hard, how often? Also there's the issue of convenience. One way to make exercise convenient is by creating your own home gym. I can hear you now: "I have no space!" and "It's too expensive." In chapter 9 I'm going to giv you a blueprint for creating a little gym in your home or office for less than a hundred dollars. The advantage, of course, to a home program is that it is an immense time-saver. You don't have to go anywhere. There's zero commute time. Plus, you can train anytime—night or day. And you don't have to compromise the integrity of your workout. All it takes is a bit of space, a few sets of dumbbells, a little time, and *doing it!*

· dumbbells mimic real-life movements ·

Some exercisers are more comfortable using machines. And machines are great for some. But one of the major drawbacks is they artificially constrain your moves.

When you pick up a dumbbell, however, it presents more of a total body challenge. It's not just about working your biceps (the front of your upper arms). Your entire musculature responds. You need a strong core and proper posture to protect your back and neck. In addition to the direct muscle group working, synergistic (helper) muscles activate in order to stabilize your back, shoulders, and legs.

Traditionally, machines work in only one plane of motion—that is, in the front, side, or back of the body. With dumbbells, you often work in two planes (biplanar) or even three (triplanar). The advantage to this is obvious, since in its normal activities your body rarely moves in a single direction at a time. Your body and limbs are transplanar—that is, they move in all directions at once in the natural world. Your axial skeleton—the bones of the head, spinal column, and chest—may be moving forward but your appendicular skeleton, consisting of your arms, shoulders, legs, and pelvis bones, may be moving side to side.

So training with dumbbells gives you not only direct strength in the muscle group you are working but overall strength through use of your stabilizing muscles.

· dumbbells force you to use proper lifting techniques ·

Proper body alignment is critical to safe and effective weight lifting. One of the advantages of machines is that, when adjusted properly, they set you up to execute moves properly. They protect your alignment, but they also limit your free range of motion. You can only go as far as the machine allows. This is both a good thing and not such a good thing. The good thing is you're fairly safe. The bad thing is your joint or body mechanics might not necessarily fit the design of the machine so they can be uncomfortable to use. I am small. (*Petite* is the politically correct term, unlike *vertically challenged*, a phrase that sort of pisses me off.) I cannot use some machines in my gym because I have to compromise my form to reach either the foot bar or the arm pads. There are some machines I can't reach at all. If you are using a piece of equipment incorrectly or if it is not right for you, you run a greater risk of injury.

When you lift dumbbells with proper form, so that your posture, body alignment, and the muscles surrounding the spine are as they should be, you protect your spine, back, and neck from injury. You have to generate your own energy as a protective mechanism. In other words, machines do some of the work for you. They don't require full-body muscle recruitment or body discipline.

· dumbbells give you training flexibility ·

Dumbbells are relatively lightweight and portable. You can pack them, move them from place to place, room to room, house to house. You can take your dumbbells with you on a business trip or vacation. You can take them to your office. This gives them a big advantage over heavy machines. Furthermore, most machines are designed to work around a single joint, and therefore only work one major muscle group at a time. That's why you have to use so many different machines in order to get a total body workout! One set of dumbbells, on the other hand, can be used to work almost every part of the body: biceps, triceps, chest, back, shoulders, legs, and butt.

· dumbbells are inexpensive ·

Creating a healthier, stronger body is not costly. You don't have to spend a lot of money and it doesn't take up a lot of space to create a home gym. In Chapter 9 I will tell you how you can create a gym that is effective, versatile, and functional for under a hundred dollars.

And here's another irresistible bargain (better than designer shoes at 75 percent off): One of the best resistance mechanisms of all is absolutely free—*your own body weight.*

Now that you know how important muscle is, in the next chapter there's information that will get you started on all the important practices you should combine with your Smart Girls program to ensure all-around fitness.

· 7 ·

. . . and seven other smart things smart girls do

· take care of your heart ·

All the knowledge I possess everyone else can acquire, but my heart is all my own.

— GOETHE

We have two hearts—well, not anatomically, unless maybe you've entered our realm from the imagination of George Lucas. But you know what I mean.

YOUR PHYSICAL HEART

First, there is your physical heart, that amazing workhorse of a muscle whose job, pumping blood throughout your body, is about as vital and un-relenting a task as you can find.

Your heart is about the size of both your fists. It beats about 100,000 times a day, 35 million times a year, and an average of 2.5 billion times in a lifetime. It is not positioned straight up and down, but sideways in your chest cavity. It has four chambers and is actually two pumps, one on the left side, one on the right. It has four valves designed to maintain blood flow in one direction. It weighs between 250 and 350 grams (although sometimes, when metaphorically broken, it feels as if it weighs a great deal more).

In addition to transporting oxygenated blood from your lungs to tissues and deoxygenated blood from the tissues back to your lungs, your heart, via your cardiovascular system—over sixty thousand miles of blood vessels—distributes nutrients, removes metabolic wastes, transports hormones and enzymes, maintains fluid volume (preventing dehydration), and helps maintain body temperature by absorbing and redistributing heat. No wonder it gets so much publicity.

The one activity for which your heart is poorly designed: *being sedentary*. It needs, indeed demands, physical activity to remain in prime working order. Like all pumps, it becomes sluggish if not used. Its capacity for circulating its *vitalis*, in this case oxygenated blood, becomes life-threateningly compromised. The healthier this fist-sized dynamo remains, the better able it is to perform its critically demanding job.

Now the "disheartening" news: Heart disease is the leading cause of death in women. We tend to develop heart disease about a decade later than men. It is believed our dear friend estrogen has heart-protective benefits that give us this grace period. As the process of menopause begins, there is a progressive decline in estrogen and with this decline emerges a complement of metabolic and physiological changes that influence your risk for heart disease: increases in weight, blood pressure, and cholesterol levels.

So how do we take care of this mighty muscle that is so unrelenting in taking care of us?

We lift (dumbbells) and *we move!*

We Lift . . .

A recent article that appeared in the *Journal of the American Medical Association* described a study that included weight-resistance training along with aerobic exercise as a physical activity to help reduce the risk of coronary heart disease. The researchers concluded that "adding weight training to the exercise program [was] among the most effective strategies to reduce the risk of CHD [coronary heart disease]." Although the study was conducted using men as subjects, future studies will explore the positive effects of weight training on lowering heart disease risk in women.

Additionally, the American Heart Association now lists weight training as one of the ways, along with a healthy diet and vigorous aerobic exercise, to lower body fat and help reduce the risk of heart disease.

. . . And We Move!

We walk or jog or do the stair stepper. We hike, we climb, we run track, we swim. We ride bikes, we dance, we jump rope. You can call it aerobics, you can call it cardio, you can call it CV (for cardiovascular). It all amounts to the same thing: increasing your heart rate by performing a steady state activity for a period of time. I gave you the prescription for cardiovascular fitness in chapter 3, but I will repeat it here once again because it is important:

FREQUENCY: All or most days of the week

INTENSITY: 60 to 90 percent of maximal heart rate

DURATION: 15 to 60 minutes

MODE: Using large muscle groups in rhythmic motion

Again, the choice of movement is up to you and what you enjoy doing. Your heart isn't particularly picky about how you're moving—swimming or walking or biking—it only cares that you're moving.

YOUR EMOTIONAL HEART

Now, on to our other heart: our emotional one. The one that leaps with excitement when something wonderful is about to happen. The one that feels as if it's breaking to bits when we experience loss or sadness or the aptly named "heartbreak." The one that poets and philosophers and saints and sages have pondered since recorded history began.

Our emotional heart is far more delicate than our muscle heart. Our

physical heart has a serious job to do. It is loath to relinquish its responsibility because a boyfriend gives us the old "I'm not ready to make a commitment," or we don't get that desired job promotion. Our emotional
heart, well, that's a whole other story. It is subject to all manner of personal
slights and injustices. Our physical heart doesn't take personally not being
asked to the prom or not getting a call or not hearing from our best friend.
It keeps pumping blood. But our emotional heart can drive us to crawl into
our beds, headfirst, with nary a backward glance when we suffer or are in
pain. Unlike the males of our species, we seem hardwired to react more
emotionally to life's Sturm und Drang.

There must be, like everything else explaining gender differences, an
evolutionary justification for this fundamental discrepancy. It might have
to do with survival adaptation.

As our cave-dwelling mates were so preoccupied with killing food, they
might not have noticed that the food was trying to kill them. Maybe our fore-
mothers' responsibility was similar to what it is today: caretaking. Maybe
their emotionality helped to protect their loved ones from potential danger
lurking outside the cave. Perhaps it was the woman's job to jump up and
down and yell, "Hey, Mooga, watch out! Woolly mammoth to your right."

Studies absolutely prove men and women's brains function on entirely
different emotional tracks. A recent study conducted in the Department of
Psychology and Radiology at Stanford University found men and women
not only express their emotions differently, they remember emotional
events in entirely different ways. The researchers reported women recall
images and experiences much more vividly than men and found them easier to recall.

Women are disproportionately affected by depression, experiencing it
at roughly twice the rate of men, according to the National Institute of
Mental Health (NIMH). The NIMH also states, "exercise is a potential
pathway to reducing depression . . . it is related to fewer depressive symptoms in observational studies and appears to be as efficacious as psy-
chotherapy in patients with mild depression."

So what does all this mean to Smart Girls? Well, when it comes to our
emotional hearts we're vulnerable (and sometimes not *that* smart). Some-

times we suffer more than we ought to and sometimes we take it out on ourselves. It is okay to feel hurt and react appropriately when sorrow, loss, or pain enters our lives. But it is never okay to treat ourselves with disdain, disrespect, or indifference.

One excellent way to take care of your emotional heart is to take care of your physical heart through exercise, whether it is going for a long walk, a bike ride, or a swim to clear your head or contemplate a troubling situation. A study conducted in the United Kingdom, which appeared in the *Journal of Sports Medicine and Physical Fitness*, reported that feelings of anger, confusion, fatigue, and tension were significantly reduced through aerobic movement. Other emotionally healing activities include long stretching with deep breathing, yoga, and meditation.

The point is, dear Smart Girls, sometimes by doing something proactive for your physical heart, your emotional heart benefits as well.

· stand tall ·

Habit, my friend, is practice long pursued, that at the last becomes the man himself.

—EVENUS

I know I told you there were no easy answers or tricky gimmicks to achieving a more beautiful physical appearance. But I lied, sort of. I do have one secret to look several pounds lighter and a few years younger, instantly!

Good posture!

Here's an experiment I'd like you to try right now. Go over to the mirror. Bend over, as if your lower back (the lumbar region) were hurting. Wince a bit. As you move, take smaller steps as if each stride sent pain shooting up into your back. Now stand up straight. Suck in your abs tightly, square off your shoulders, maintain a straight spine, and move with conviction, strength, and fluidity. Good posture.

Can't you see the difference immediately? Just sucking in your abdominals and standing up straight gives a slimmer appearance. Turn sideways and check it out. And you can do this anytime you choose. Sloppy body carriage has nothing to do with what we eat, how much we weigh, or exercise. *It's a reflection of how we feel about ourselves and our sense of personal pride.*

Sometimes poor posture is the result of some congenital weakness in a person's skeletal structure. But sometimes it's the result of laziness, stress, or even lack of body awareness.

Below are some common causes of poor posture:

- Weak muscles
- Injuries
- Poor nutrition
- Foot problems
- Stress
- Low self-esteem
- Subluxation (partial dislocation in a joint)
- Poor eyesight
- Being overweight
- Abdominal fat
- Pregnancy
- Poor quality or soft mattresses
- Self-consciousness about one's height

TEST YOUR POSTURE

You can test your posture right now by doing the wall test. Health practitioners often use this procedure to evaluate postural alignment and areas of structural weakness in the axial and appendicular skeleton.

Stand with the back of your head, shoulder blades, and buttocks against a wall and your heels two to four inches from the wall. In this position, your hand should fit snugly between your lower back and the wall. If there is too much space between the wall and your lumbar (lower back)—that is, if it is wider than the thickness of your hand, adjust your posture forward by tightening your abdominal wall and shifting your pelvis to decrease the space. If you can't squeeze your hand between your lower back and the wall, then tighten your abdominals and shift your pelvic bone backward to increase the space between your lower back and wall.

The test should give you a good evaluation of what correct posture looks and feels like. If you have a spinal defect, such as scoliosis (curvature of the spine), you will be limited by how you can physically adjust your posture on your own. If you have or suspect you have some spinal misalignment, disc or vertebral problems, or injury causing you chronic pain, joint and neck problems, limited range of motion, or fatigue, then consult your physician for a complete evaluation.

Two extreme forms of poor posture are kyphosis and lordosis. Kyphosis is holding your body in such a way that your shoulders roll forward and your chest muscles are foreshortened. In other words, slouching. Lordosis is commonly referred to as being "swaybacked." Structurally, it is when your stomach sticks out too far in front of you and your buttocks sticks out too far behind, which results in an extreme curve between the pelvic bone and the ribs of the lumbar region. These types of postural weaknesses can be improved significantly by practicing good posture.

You're probably thinking this is easier said than done. One more thing to add to your already growing list of daily personal chores and responsibilities. But wait! Practicing good posture is simply a matter of choice. It produces extraordinary results with minimal physical or emotional effort, no extra time expenditure, and zero cost. It is a great new habit to learn. Good posture sends out a positive and profound message to the world: I have self-esteem. I take pride in my being. I am important. All that, dear Smart Girls, just by *standing tall.*

· stretch your body:
the stretch recipes ·

Stretch your foot to the length of your blanket.

— PERSIAN PROVERB

The primary physical goals of a comprehensive stretching program are to maintain the full range of motion around joints, prevent lower back and neck injury, and maintain elasticity in the connective tissues. But stretching also helps create long, lean muscle. It helps you relax and reduce stress. It can even help you sleep better. Some additional benefits of stretching include:

- Maintaining flexibility for everyday activities
- Maintaining and enhancing joint range of motion
- Reducing risk of exercise-related injuries
- Reducing muscular soreness
- Enhancing overall body awareness
- Increasing ability to achieve physical relaxation

A suitable stretching program is a critical component to your overall physical conditioning as well as your general health.

TYPES OF STRETCHES:

STATIC STRETCHING	Long, slow stretches in which you hold the stretch for ten seconds or more.
DYNAMIC STRETCHING	Controlled leg and arm movements that take you gently to the limits of your range of motion.
ACTIVITY-SPECIFIC STRETCHING	Stretches targeted to warm up muscle groups and increase range of motion

PASSIVE STRETCHING

in a joint area to be used for exercise or sports.

Also called relaxed stretch, these are ones in which you are assisted by either a partner or equipment (i.e., a towel, surgical tubing) to execute the stretch.

HOW TO STRETCH CORRECTLY

- Never vigorously stretch cold muscles. Always warm up two to five minutes by walking, taking a warm shower, or turning on the car heater on the way to the gym, especially on chilly mornings.
- Stretch slowly, and release the breath as you move into or deepen the stretch.
- Do not bounce or force stretches.
- Hold stretches for ten to thirty seconds.
- When you are in the deepest part of the stretch, exhale into it, relaxing muscles throughout the movement.

hamstring hug

●—●

This is a stretch that can be done by most everyone, regardless of fitness level, age, or gender. It stretches the muscles of the back of the leg (the hamstring muscles). The hamstring group comprises three muscles that are primarily responsible for flexing your knee and secondarily for extending your hip. Tight or inflexible hamstring muscles are often the cause of low back pain.

* Lie on your back on a firm surface, preferably the floor, to protect your spine.
* Place your hands between the knee and the foot of one leg, not on the knee itself, and not behind your leg right on the hamstrings.
* Gently bring the knee toward your chest, hugging it tightly.
* If you have any low back pain or discomfort, bend the knee of the nonworking leg (the leg not being stretched), keeping your foot on the floor.
* Don't worry about how close your knee comes to your chest. Everyone's level of flexibility is different.
* Do the Hamstring Hug first one leg at a time and then both legs together.

the lumbar twist

This stretch is ideal for releasing tightness and tension in the lower back region, a particularly vulnerable area for most people. It is one of those stretches that feels so good, you wonder why you don't do it more often.

- Lie on your back, both legs straight out in front.
- Bring one knee toward your chest as you would do for the Hamstring Hug.
- Drop the knee across the nonworking straight leg.
- Using the hand opposite the bent knee, press the crossed-over leg gently toward the floor.
- Stretch your other arm and bring it out in line with your shoulder, pressing your back into the floor. This gives your spine a long stretch.
- Release leg slowly and repeat on the other side.

stretch recipe #2

lateral waist bends

This is an excellent upper torso, back, and oblique stretch. It can be done either standing or seated on the floor in an open-legged position.

- If you are standing, place your feet hip-distance apart. If you are seated on the floor, bring your legs out in an open leg straddle to your comfort level.
- Contract your abdominals, stand or sit up straight, and feel as if you are pulling yourself up tall, out of your ribs.
- Bring your hands behind your head, elbows sticking out sideways.
- Leading with one elbow, slowly stretch by bending down toward that side. If you are standing, do not allow your hips to shift from side to side.
- As your elbow drops down, you should feel a stretch in your lats (back) and across your ribs in front and in the obliques.
- Return to your starting position and stretch to the other side.

head and neck rotations

The muscles of the neck and head are some of the least used in full range of motion activities. You just don't think about using these muscles in a concentrated way and eventually, as you age, your range of motion becomes shorter and shorter. In addition to protecting your range of motion, these exercises help release tension in the neck and upper back, can help relieve headache symptoms, and are helpful for general relaxation. They can be performed virtually anywhere (except while driving, please!).

* Sit up or stand tall, abdominals tucked in.
* Start with your head straight, eyes forward, shoulders relaxed. Chin should not be tucked under or head hyperextended.
* Keeping your head level, slowly rotate it to one side, bringing the chin over your shoulder as close as possible but without dropping the chin down.
* Hold the head in that position for just about three seconds and then slowly rotate over to the other shoulder, still keeping your head level.
* Do ten to fifteen rotations three times a day, or more if you are feeling tense or stressed.

stretch recipe #4

shoulder rolls

Along with Head and Neck Rotations, Shoulder Rolls help to relieve tension in the neck, back, and shoulders, areas that are most vulnerable to stress. Again, these are simple exercises that can be performed anywhere.

- Sit up or stand tall, abdominals contracted.
- Gently rotate your shoulders back, bringing them close to your ears; then, as they drop, squeeze the shoulder blades (the scapulae) as close together as possible.
- After you do twelve rear shoulder rolls, reverse the movement for twelve front rolls—bring your shoulders up then forward, shortening your chest muscles.
- Do the movements slowly, along with easy breathing; to enhance the concentration, close your eyes and feel the muscles move and relax.
- Also, as you're doing these, try to let the tension release all over your body, neck, spine, and lower back.

stretch recipe #5

seated inner thigh stretch

This stretch focuses primarily on stretching the inner thighs, but as your flexibility increases, you will also feel a nice stretch in the lower back.

- Sit on the floor and bring the soles of your feet together far enough away from your body so the space forms a diamond shape.
- Start this stretch by sitting up tall and contracting your abdominal wall.
- Take a deep inhalation and as you exhale, slowly drop your chest over your feet.
- Try and push your knees toward the floor so you feel the deep stretch in your inner thigh areas. You can do this by gently pressing your knees down using your hands. But do not bounce your knees.
- Hang down over your knees for about thirty to forty-five seconds.
- Roll back up, one vertebra at a time, into the tall, seated position.

stretch recipe #6

piriformis stretch

●—●

The piriformis is one of the six deep-lateral rotator muscles located at the hip. They are the muscles responsible for externally rotating the hip. Strengthening and stretching the piriformis and surrounding muscles helps prevent pain in the hip and buttocks that can radiate up into the lower back and leg and may help in protecting against a severe form of nerve damage called sciatica.

- Lying on your back on a supportive surface, knees up, cross one leg over the thigh of the other leg just as you would if you were seated in a chair crossing your leg over.
- Lift the bottom leg off the ground, using it as leverage to push the crossed leg toward your chest.
- You will feel a gentle stretch on the outside of your buttocks.
- If you want to deepen the stretch, place your hands around the calf or ankle of the uncrossed leg and pull it toward you.
- Lower the leveraging leg's foot to the ground and then lift up again.
- Execute the movements slowly and with control. Don't throw the leg up and down.
- Do ten to fifteen repetitions on one side and then repeat on the other side.

· general stretch prescription ·

DURATION	FREQUENCY	TECHNIQUE
Hold each stretch 10–30 seconds	3–6 times a week	Slow, static stretches— no bouncing. Release breath slowly through the stretch.

· have fun ·

Isn't fun the best thing to have?

—FROM THE MOVIE *ARTHUR*

Remember when you were a little girl and playing outside—running, skipping, jumping—wasn't work, it was play? And it was fun. Far more fun than being anchored to a desk trying to put to memory the details of the Battle of Hastings or the periodic table. What happened?

One way to increase the exercise fun factor is to train with a friend or partner. There are many mornings (more than I would like to admit) when my alarm goes off at four thirty (yes, that's A.M.) and the last thing I want to do is leave the warmth and comfort of my snug bed to cozy up to the hard, cold reality of dumbbells. But I know Mitchell, my training partner, will be waiting for me. So two things are in play: first, I've made a commitment and I feel some accountability. If I said I'd be at the gym at five o'clock and he's waiting for me at five o'clock, I'd feel awful if I were a no-show. Second, Mitchell makes me laugh. So every morning at five o'clock I'm laughing. Even if initially I don't feel like working out, I can't think of a better way to start the day than by laughing.

It is also important to find fun and pleasure in other activities in your life as well. Attitude is everything. "Feeling joy" is an underrated pursuit. It seems self-indulgent and frivolous. But have you ever looked at the face of someone who is experiencing joy and happiness in what they are doing? They possess an undeniable glow and effervescence.

A recent study conducted at Stanford University revealed that the brain responds to happy expressions, such as smiling, but only in people who are open to receiving positive emotions. Through MRI imaging the researchers discovered that the amygdala, the region of the brain responsible for arousal, responds positively primarily in people who are extroverts.

This is a sort of game I play while I am on my aerobic walks around my neighborhood. When I am approaching someone and I see they are not smiling, I smile at them. Ninety-nine percent of the time the person smiles back. And I think to myself how much more attractive that person looks with that smile. I know this all sounds quite Pollyanna-ish, and it sort of is, except that we spend hundreds of billions of dollars (not individually, of course, although sometimes it sure feels like it) on cosmetics, cosmetic procedures, creams, salves, and surgery for our physical enhancement. I'm not saying smiling is a replacement for taking care of your skin or hair or body, but a smile is a built-in beautifier. Promise!

· eat wise but don't deny ·

Tell me what you eat and I will tell you who you are.

—ANTHELME BRILLAT-SAVARIN

What's interesting about we humans is how we can convert a basic and vital biological need into a complicated matrix of myths, ideologies, dogma, political platforms, fears, fantasies, and frustrations. We're the only animals that do so. Our other planetmates simply eat to survive and function. It's all fairly simple. And yet, in our modernized Western culture, we've elevated this life-sustaining necessity into one of the most controversial, daunting, and incendiary issues of our times.

I have some thoughts about nutrition, but I am not a dietitian. If you need help designing a diet for weight management, if you are suffering from any kind of eating disorder or disordered eating, or if you have been diagnosed with any metabolic disease, you should seek the help of a registered dietitian. When my patients or clients ask for help designing their diets, I refer them to a registered dietitian, not a nutritionist. Here's the difference: A registered dietitian must go through a rigorous academic course and accreditation process, including a supervised internship with a minimum of nine hundred hours, while anyone can call herself a nutritionist. It is ambiguous, sort of one of those hang-out-your-shingle catchphrases requiring no certification. This is not to say that there might not be some very knowledgeable nutritionists, but for the most part, you are much safer in the hands of a registered dietitian.

If you need help finding an R.D., you can log on to www.eatright.org; the website for the American Dietetic Association. It offers a link to finding a dietitian in your area, plus other very valuable information on nutrition.

My personal feeling about diet is this: Keep it clean and keep it lean. And sometimes, yeah, go for the fun. I mean this seriously. If you can regulate your diet most of the time, by eating lean proteins such as fish, chicken, and turkey; lots of fresh fruits and vegetables; and other high-fiber, unprocessed, low-fat foods, hey, you're doing a great job. And then sometimes, yeah baby, Mr. Cheesecake is coming your way. My food Achilles tendon is guacamole. Set a bowl of guacamole in front of me and I'll eat it like a bowl of ice cream. Occasionally I allow myself the indulgence. But then, without incrimination, I go back to my more spartan and self-disciplined ways without the feelings of deprivation that cause so many of us to fall headfirst off our carefully constructed diet wagon.

Another food I can't keep in the house is potato chips. I will eat the entire bag. So if my son insists on having some chips in the house and I find them (sometimes I make him hide them from me), I count out the ten I allot myself and put them in a plastic baggy and that gives me some sense of control plus a reality check on the amount of calories I am actually consuming. Pretzels, chips (even baked ones), peanuts, crackers, cereal—all these dry food items I call "fist foods." They're treacherous because you can eat them by the fistful without a second's thought, and before you know it you've consumed several hundred calories without feeling you've eaten anything at all.

· wear properly fitted
exercise shoes ·

It is better to wear out than to rust out.

— RICHARD CUMBERLAND

I am frequently asked, "What is the best piece of aerobic equipment I can buy?" My answer to this is unequivocal: The single best piece of exercise equipment you can own is *a good pair of shoes.*

You may own a three-thousand-dollar treadmill, but if you're jogging or walking on improperly fitted shoes, trouble is just a stride away.

What makes a good shoe? Is price an indicator of quality? What is a proper fit? Do they have to be expensive to be good? How long should a pair of shoes last?

In search of the answers to these FAQs, I asked the smartest man I know in the business of fitting athletic shoes. His name is Charlie Hoover. As his first sport, he was a long-distance cyclist. Then he became a marathon runner. He owns and operates the best athletic shoe store in Los Angeles. He and his staff are brilliant and tireless at the art of properly fitting athletic shoes. They take it very seriously. He named his store in honor of the first marathon runner, an indefatigable Athenian, Phidippides.

Following is some of our interview:

J: *When buying shoes, how does one know if they're being properly fitted?*

C: There should be about a finger's width between the longest toe and the front of the shoe. There is a limited availability of widths so this fitting formula could result in some shoes being too wide. Obviously, compromises may be necessary and you need to determine how short the shoes can be without losing your toenails. The lacebox sides should be parallel to each other, not in an open or inverted "V." The slack across the ball of the foot should be minimal, and there should be no excess pressure diagonally from the ball of the big toe to the "ball" joint of the little toe. Heel slippage should be minimal. Again, this is highly subjective.

J: *What should a woman look for in a good shoe?*

C: Most people—75 to 80 percent of the population—overpronate, that is, their feet turn outward with a raising of the outside edge. Stability is the most important quality to look for in a shoe. The more stable shoes tend to be firmer. The heel counter (the part that holds the heel) should be firm and well anchored (preferably with a reinforcing collar) to the midsole—commonly the white squishy part of the shoe. The shoe should flex easily at the ball of the foot. Shoes that bend in the middle (and there are a lot of them out there!) should be avoided. Such shoes are an invitation for disaster. Sole material is largely a matter of preference. Hard heel strikers or folks who wear out the forefoot quickly need to stick to high-abrasion rubber materials. The upper material should be breathable. Larger gauge mesh generally wears better than smaller gauge, especially on trails, where the grit acts as an abrasive.

J: *What about cost? Are more expensive shoes better?*

C: Definitely not. But it is hard these days to find a decent shoe with a good set of features under sixty five dollars. The average price is between seventy-five and eighty-five dollars. Shoes that cost twice as much will *not* last twice as long. I myself usually wear a running shoe that costs about eighty dollars.

J: *How long should shoes last?*

C: Most people will never actually *wear out* their shoes. The support and cushioning will go long before the shoe is "worn out." Body weight, biomechanics, running surface, and weather all affect how long shoes will last. Most males below 180 pounds with no biome-chanical problems can go about 500 miles on a shoe. Females usually weigh less and will, on average, go about 150 miles longer on a shoe.

J: *What is the difference between the various shoes: running, walking, cross-trainers?*

c: Walking shoes should, in fact, be somewhat different from running shoes, but due to the marketing positioning of walking shoes, there are *very* few that can hold a candle to even a medium-support-level running shoe. Most walking shoes are built to appeal aesthetically to the market that is looking for them: not too bulky, done in white leather, nice clean looks, so forth. Unfortunately, this usually trans-lates into a shoe that is not very supportive. Cross-trainers combine some running shoe features with court shoe features and are appro-priate choices for someone doing a bit of everything.

J: *What advice can you give about how to shop for proper athletic shoes?*

c: Try to shop somewhere where the salespeople know what they are doing. They need to know their shoes, know a fair amount about bio-mechanics and fit. Preferably, they should be runners themselves. It's kind of hard to trust someone talking about running shoes who smells like cigarettes. Bring your old shoes with you. It helps to look at wear patterns. Remember, there is often a huge gulf between what a manufacturer *says* about a shoe and who it is for, versus how the shoe actually performs! The less running and shoe experience you have, the more of an experiment each shoe purchase is. Try to make the best of failed experiences. Learn from mistakes and make a bet-ter choice the next time.

Try to make the best of failed experiences. Learn from mistakes and make a better choice the next time. Sounds like good advice from Charlie. In or out of the shoe store.

· care for yourself physically and emotionally ·

Now I know the things I know,
And do the things I do;
And if you do not like me so,
To Hell, my love, with you!

— DOROTHY PARKER

The underlying theme of *Smart Girls Do Dumbbells* is about taking care of yourself, *completely*. The Smart Girls dumbbell program is a sound and sensible program for strengthening your body, protecting your health, and becoming physically self-aware. But also, and equally important, it's about taking care of your emotional self and your personal well-being. Because becoming physically strong has amazing ramifications. Physical strength translates into personal power, a sense of accomplishment, and self-respect.

These emotional strengths don't just stay in the gym. You carry these hard-earned attributes with you to other aspects of your life as well. When you feel a sense of physical pride, your sense of personal pride escalates exponentially.

We often feel selfish or undeserving when it comes to caring for ourselves. We take tremendous pride (as well we should) in being good mothers, wives, daughters, sisters, friends. It is a primary focus for a lot of us. We often sacrifice our needs to tend to others.

I work once a week with a woman named Charlotte. She is diabetic and overweight. When she first came to see me, she walked with a cane because of her severely arthritic knee and ankle joints. During the consultation we talked for quite a while about her goals and expectations. She had an elderly mother for whom she cared, a business she was responsible for, and a large extended family she supported financially.

"Of course I want to lose this weight. That's the most important thing. But, also, I need to take time for myself, to take care of myself. Making this commitment to come work with you is a priority for me. I have always put everyone else before myself and now I am a mess physically, and my health is suffering. It's time to start taking care of me!"

Charlotte's resolve has paid off. Several months after starting her exercise program she is able to walk unassisted. She no longer requires her oral insulin and she is slowly losing some of her weight.

HOW SMART GIRLS TAKE CARE OF THEMSELVES PHYSICALLY

- Drink 6 to 8 eight-ounce glasses of water a day.
- Wear sunblock every day.
- Do not smoke.
- Do self–breast examinations.
- Have annual physical checkups.
- Take care of your bones by getting enough calcium through food or supplements.
- Floss your teeth!

SMART GIRLS TAKE CARE OF THEMSELVES EMOTIONALLY

- Don't be hard on yourself if you miss a day of exercise, or if you eat something that is not on your diet.
- Do something that brings you pure and utter joy and acknowledge it by saying, "This is giving me pure and utter joy."
- Never allow anyone to make you feel "less than."
- Surround yourself with people who respect you.
- Surround yourself with people whom you respect.
- Take pride in your accomplishments and never underestimate your abilities.
- Laugh at least once a day (and hopefully more!).

· 8 ·

can't forget
those abs!

ah, abs! The eternal struggle for flat, sleek, bikini-wearing abs. Be
gone the lower pouch. The jeans that don't zip. The below-the-belt
bloat.

But are firm abdominals the province of real women in the real world?
Or are they some idealized form of the female body, impossible for mortals
to achieve? The answer is yes . . . and no. Most of us don't possess the physiology, genetics, or just plain good luck to achieve the ab perfection of
swimsuit models.

The good news is, however, it is certainly within your power to achieve
firmer, stronger abs. The ultimate goal for Smart Girls is to create the ideal
abdominal structure for *your body type* consistent with your fitness and
health needs.

And do not worry that the quest for strong abdominals is in the name
of vanity alone. One of the main reasons to incorporate a well-designed abdominal program into your regular workout routine is to increase your
core strength for a healthier back and spine. A strong core and abdominals help protect your back, as well as relieve low back pain. In a report
commissioned by Congress, the National Academy of Science revealed that

low back pain contributes to around $50 billion in medical costs, patient care, and lost earnings annually.

Strong abdominals help you create and maintain good posture that protects the spine, shoulders, and neck. I talked about posture in some detail in chapter 7, but it is worth mentioning here again because 80 percent of Americans experience low back pain, and poor posture is a contributing factor.

· ab anatomy ·

You may imagine your abdominal section as just one big muscle, but it's not. It is actually five muscles: the rectus abdominis, external and internal obliques, transversus abdominis, and quadratus abdominis.

The rectus abdominis, the major muscle located in the midsection of your trunk, is a very long muscle that begins at the crest of the pubis and inserts at the cartilage of the fifth, sixth, and seventh ribs. It is the muscle that controls the tilt of the pelvic region and, by extension, the curvature of the lower spine. That is why weak abdominal muscles are directly correlated to lower back problems.

The external and internal obliques are located on either side of the rectus abdominis. The transversus abdominis is located in the lower region of the abdominal wall, around the hips and toward the pelvic region.

The muscles of the abdominals assist in flexing the trunk of the body. For instance, when you bend down to touch your toes, the action of the abs is flexion. Your internal and external obliques come into play during lateral motion—side moves—like twisting. The transversus abdominis muscle activates during forced exhalation by pulling the abdominal inward, as in an Isometric Contraction.

the
ab exercise
recipes

isometric contractions

target: the core—transversus abdominis

Isometric Contractions are the ideal way to exercise the transversus abdominis muscle, a stabilizing and core-strengthening muscle. What's wonderful about these Isometric Contractions is that they can be performed anywhere, seated or standing, at work, at your desk, waiting in line for a film or at a checkout stand. Simply contract the abdominal wall, pulling back as tightly as possible. Hold the contraction from fifteen to sixty seconds. It is especially important to begin all the exercises that follow by first doing Isometric Contractions. Another easy way to fit in a little extra ab work is to isometrically contract your abs while you're doing your aerobics, walking, jogging, or using a stair climber. And here's a nice bonus: Focusing on this muscle group by keeping it tight and contracted benefits your posture as well. It's almost an automatic reflex—tighten your abs, and suddenly you're standing taller, pulling back your shoulders, and holding your head higher. Try it!

reverse leg lifts

target: lower regions of the abs

Lying on your back, place your hands under the small of your back. This helps protect the lower (lumbar) region of the spine by stabilizing it and preventing hyperextension. Place legs and feet together with a slight bend in the knees. Moving legs in unison, keeping feet together and knees slightly bent, bring the legs toward the chest. Do not allow the body to rock with the momentum of the movement, but slowly, smoothly pull the thighs in, *contracting the abs,* and then slowly, smoothly bring the legs back parallel to, but not touching, the floor. Feel the lengthening action of the movement.

ab exercise recipe #2

torso twists

●—●

target: external and internal obliques

The Torso Twist targets the waist muscles—external and internal obliques. Lie on your back and bend your knees to 90 degrees and place your feet either on the floor or on a bed or chair. You can also cross one leg over the other. Put your hands behind your head, and lift your upper body off the ground so your shoulders do not touch the floor—this is the starting and ending position. Twist the trunk by moving one elbow toward the opposite knee, bringing it as close to the knee as possible, without pulling on your neck or compromising your form by lifting your back off the ground. If you look straight up at the ceiling, this will help keep your body in alignment and prevent you from hurting your neck or doing the Torso Twist incorrectly. Repeat to the other side. Doing it once on each side constitutes one repetition.

traditional crunches

●—●

target: upper regions of the abs

For beginners, place the hands across the chest; this prevents you from pulling on the neck. If you are more advanced, place your hands behind your head. For the highly advanced, your arms can be extended above the head, parallel to the ears. Lying on your back, place your feet on a chair, bed, or bench, the floor, or perpendicular to the floor with feet crossed at the ankles. Lift the shoulders slightly off the floor; they should not touch the floor as you execute the move or between repetition. The trick to executing the Crunch correctly is moving the entire upper body as a unit, head aligned with the spine. As you move the body upward, lead with your chest, eyes facing upward toward the ceiling remembering to *keep the abs contracted* throughout the entire rep. Your back does not lift off the floor. And breathe! Now this is critical: As you release the Crunch, moving back to the starting position, hold the contraction, feel the lengthening action, and do not allow your shoulders to hit the mat or touch the floor.

combo crunches

●—●

target: lower and upper abdominals

If you are in a time crunch, Combo Crunches work both the lower and the upper abdominal areas simultaneously. Lie on the floor and bring the legs perpendicular to the torso, crossing the feet at the ankles. Place your hands behind your head. Again, remember to protect your neck by not pulling on it. Shoulders do not rest on the floor or mat. Your elbows point toward your knees. In this move, bring the upper body toward the legs as the legs are lifting and the hips are curling and contracting inward, allowing the elbows to meet with and touch the knees. If your knees and elbows don't touch, that's okay . . . mainly concentrate on the crunch of both the upper and the lower abdominals.

pelvic tilts

●—●

target: lower abdominals and muscles of the pelvic floor

Pelvic Tilts are a great lower abdominal alternative to Leg Lifts. They work the muscle fibers of the lower abs in a highly focused, isometric move that isolates the lower abdominals without being overly aggressive on the lumbar area if you suffer from a weak lower back or if Reverse Curls are too difficult. As the name implies, they also work the muscles of the pelvic floor, similar to Kegel exercises, which were developed by Dr. Arnold Kegel to help women control urinary problems.

Pelvic Tilts are best done on the floor using your exercise mat to cushion your back and protect your spine. Lying on the floor, hands resting at your sides, bend your knees and place your feet on the floor about fifteen inches in front of your buttocks. Make certain your feet are parallel and facing forward.

Gently tilt your hips up but *without arching your back.* If your back is too arched, you are hyperextending the lower back and this is not the correct position.

With your buttocks no more than five or six inches off the mat, isometrically contract the abdominals. With each contraction, it should feel as if you are "curling" your lower abs toward you. You will also be squeezing your buttocks at the same time, but don't let the buttocks take over the work of the abdominals.

ab exercise recipe #6

· don't forget to breathe! ·

Just because you've contracted the abdominal wall doesn't mean you should stop breathing! This is a very common reflex for those who are not used to breathing properly as they exercise—whether you're doing your dumbbell exercises or your abdominal work.

Holding your breath during exercise is called the Valsalva maneuver, which is an expiratory effort against a closed glottis. The glottis is the narrowest part of the larynx through which air passes into and out of the trachea. The Valsalva maneuver increases pressure within the thoracic (chest) cavity and thereby interferes with venous return of blood to the heart.

It takes some practice to get your breathing and body movements working in concert. Take some time to focus on your breathing rhythms as you exercise, and soon it will become an automatic reflex.

· six abdominal exercise recipes ·

	BEGINNER		INTERMEDIATE		ADVANCED	
	SETS	REPS	SETS	REPS	SETS	REPS
Recipe #1 ISOMETRIC CONTRACTIONS (Note: These can be done at one time or throughout the day.)	2–5	Hold for 15 seconds	5–10	Hold for 15–30 seconds	10–15	Hold for 30–60 seconds
Recipe #2 REVERSE LEG LIFTS	2	5–10	3	10–15	3	15–25
Recipe #3 TORSO TWISTS	2	5–10	3	10–15	3	15–25
Recipe #4 TRADITIONAL CRUNCHES	2	5–10	3	10–15	3	15–25
Recipe #5 COMBO CRUNCHES	2	5–10	3	10–20	3	20–25
Recipe #6 PELVIC TILTS	2	15–20	3	20–25	3	25–30

building your personalized dumbbell gym (for under $100)

"**i** haven't done my dumbbell exercises since we worked out last," Ryan tells me. It's been nearly a month since I last saw her.

"What's been going on?" I ask.

"I just couldn't get it together to exercise. I had to gather old clothes for a garage sale. Then my sister came to visit from New Hampshire and I had to spend time with her. She broke up with her boyfriend. Plus her cat is missing. She's depressed."

"You should have brought her with you today! She would have felt better after we worked out."

"Oh, she left three weeks ago."

"Three weeks ago! So what happened to you in the meantime?"

"Oh, I dunno."

"Maybe you got out of the groove?" I offered. "The days slipped away? Before you knew it, you forgot to prioritize your exercise. By the time you remembered, the day was over and it was too late to go to the gym. Any of this sound possible?"

"All of it. And I could give you some more if you're interested. The more I didn't exercise the easier it was not to exercise. It's just that sometimes the *going* is harder than the *doing*, if you know what I mean."

Oh yes, I knew exactly what she meant.

And probably you do, too. I rarely hear anyone I work with complain about the actual *physical* act of working out. In fact, most of the women I work with are quite excited about how they feel while doing their dumbbell exercises and especially when they're finished with their session! It is not unusual to hear exuberant comments more along the lines of, "I feel so much better now. I love to feel my muscles working. I'm so glad I worked out."

If the stumbling block is not the working out itself, then what is it? Actually, as I've said, there is a whole host of "whatisits?" that, keep us, unlike the mail carriers, from our appointed rounds. One of the leading factors predicting our ability to exercise regularly is *convenience*.

If you have to travel too far or too long, if the gym or exercise facility is difficult to get to, if the parking is out of the way or costly, if you don't feel safe, if it is dark or if the weather is bad and you don't want to go out—all of these inconveniences will seriously impede your ability to work out on a consistent basis. (There's no tricking me. I know that if you have the tiniest excuse not to exercise, you'll use it.) Not that you're lazy, it's just as Ryan said, *getting to* the exercise is often harder than *doing* the exercise! What's the solution then?

A home gym.

You're probably thinking, "What! A home gym? I don't have the money or the space. I'm not a rock star. I'm a teacher (nurse/writer/executive assistant/salesperson/veterinarian/mother . . .). A home gym is a luxury."

Well, you may not be a rock star (yet) but you can definitely create a workout area to call your own, and it does not have to take a lot of space or a lot of money, and it's not a luxury because when it comes to your health it is a *necessity*.

· what will i need to get started? ·

Following is your basic home gym shopping list:

1. Dumbbells—two or three sets
2. Exercise mat
3. Mirror
4. Towels—one large, one hand-sized
5. Step stool

DUMBBELLS

Dumbbells are also called free weights. They come in a variety of forms and prices, ranging from as low as forty-four cents a pound for iron to two dollars a pound for chrome. The material you choose is up to you. Consider how they feel in your hand and what appeals to you aesthetically. I recommend vinyl (neoprene)–coated ones for both their comfort and their visual appeal, as they often come in a variety of attractive colors: purple, green, yellow, red.

· the beauty of dumbbells ·

When I speak of the beauty of dumbbells I'm sure you realize I am not talking about their physical appearance as much as their functional beauty (although these days dumbbells come in a delightful array of splashy colors and a wide range of sizes to meet all fitness levels).

I want to take a moment here to remind you of our discussion in chapter 6 on why dumbbells are the ideal exercise equipment.

1. Results
2. Convenience

3. Muscles used as in real-world activities
4. Force you to use proper lifting techniques
5. Training flexibility
6. Affordability

This is what I mean by the beauty of dumbbells. No other piece of resistance exercise equipment offers you this flexibility and opportunity. Single-jointed machines (the type of equipment normally found in commercial gyms and fitness centers) are large, heavy pieces of equipment, requiring a lot of space, and they are out of reach of most of our budgets. This is not the case with dumbbells, however. They're egalitarian as well as utilitarian.

· not a room of one's own ·

"And where am I going to find the space?" you say. None to spare, right? You live in a studio apartment, a college dorm room, a house you share with a roommate, or your kids have their toys all over the place and there's your husband's large-screen plasma TV taking up every last bit of space in the family room. So where do I suggest you make this little dumbbell gym of yours? *Anywhere!*

What makes dumbbells so wonderful is that even ones that weigh twenty-five or forty-five pounds don't take up a lot of space. They're compact by design. A set of six dumbbells can fit into a small corner of your closet, bedroom, living room, anywhere! But a word of advice: Select an area that is convenient. The space you recruit for your dumbbells should be a place where you have easy access, enough space to do your exercises comfortably and properly, and adequate ventilation. If you have to drag the dumbbells out from somewhere and place them somewhere else, it becomes inconvenient. If they are in full view, just waiting for you to pay them some attention, it is far easier to get started. There's an old saying, usually reserved for romantic situations but equally applicable here: Out of sight, out of mind. You'll want to keep your dumbbells front and center—or at least in a convenient corner.

· anatomy of a dumbbell ·

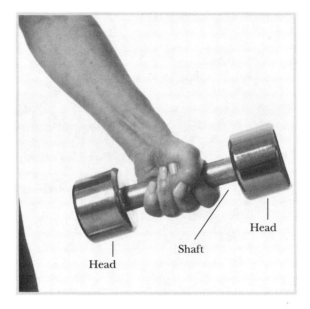

Head

Shaft

Head

The origin of the word *dumbbells* comes from the practice of removing clappers from bells, rendering them soundless during lifting.

· typical neoprene dumbbell prices ·

SIZE	PER DUMBBELL	PER SET OF TWO
1 lb.	$0.95	$1.90
2 lb.	1.95	3.90
3 lb.	2.95	5.90

SIZE	PER DUMBBELL	PER SET OF TWO
4 lb.	3.95	7.90
5 lb.	4.95	9.90
6 lb.	5.95	11.90
7 lb.	6.95	13.90
8 lb.	7.95	15.90
9 lb.	8.95	17.90
10 lb.	9.95	19.90

Some exercisers prefer outfitting the gym with chrome dumbbells because they're the type most frequently used in commercial gym facilities. However, they tend to be a little bit more expensive than neoprene and also don't come in the incremental sizes.

· typical chrome dumbbell prices ·

SIZE	PER SET OF TWO
3 lb.	$11.40
5 lb.	19.00
8 lb.	30.40

SIZE	PER SET OF TWO
10 lb.	38.00
12 lb.	45.60
15 lb.	57.00
20 lb.	76.00

As I said, what size dumbbells you select is totally dependent upon your fitness level and goals. Some women start off using five-pound dumbbells, where others find two-pound dumbbells significantly challenging. As a general rule with most of the women I work with, I have found that a basic beginning set usually consists of a pair each of three-, five-, and eight-pounders.

If we assume these denominations are your basic beginning set, the cost of your dumbbell equipment comes out to around thirty-two dollars.

Before you buy *any* equipment, I suggest you go first to an established gym or exercise facility and test your strength with their equipment. Selecting the correct dumbbell sizes for your strength and fitness level is discussed in chapter 10. As a little preview of the advice coming up ahead, I will tell you this: You can never go wrong by *starting low and going slow!*

EXERCISE MAT

An exercise mat is the next most valuable piece of equipment you can use in your workout area. One of my favorite styles of mat has a core of poly-foam, about two inches thick, covered in heavy vinyl with heavy nylon stitching. I like it because it is lightweight, easy to carry, and durable, and it provides good support for your back, neck, and spine for any floor work, abdominal exercises, and stretch routines. A good, supportive mat is especially necessary if your exercise space has hardwood flooring or another type of ungiving surface.

Additionally, the vinyl covering makes it easy to wipe down and is mildew resistant as well. A good utilitarian size is two feet by six feet (and two inches thick), which costs around forty dollars.

Another popular type of mat is a yoga-style mat, which is made of soft, durable material and provides a nonslip surface for stretching and yoga postures. They are much thinner than the exercise mat described above, measuring only about one-eighth inch thick. They're also less costly, averaging around nineteen dollars. I prefer the thicker-style polyfoam mats, if you're not doing yoga, because of the support they provide for the spine, back, and neck.

MIRROR

Watching yourself perform the dumbbell exercises gives you vital visual feedback so you can:

1. Learn proper form
2. Monitor your technique
3. Take pride in your results
4. Stay motivated

You can buy a little wood-framed full-length mirror for about nine dollars in a hardware store.

If you don't have a full-length mirror in the area you are recruiting for your workout space, don't worry about it. When I work with people in their homes, they don't always have mirrors, so sometimes we just use the reflection from the television screen. When you are just starting to use your dumbbells, you can go into a room with a mirror just to check and see if you are lifting the dumbbells correctly. After a while it will become second nature so you won't always need the visual feedback. But it is fun . . . and quite a nice little ego-booster and motivator when you see those beautiful muscles developing and working!

TOWELS

I know towels seem like pretty basic household items you can grab at any time. But it's a good idea to buy or designate towels that will remain exclusively in your workout area. I recommend two different sizes: a large bath towel to cover your exercise mat and a hand towel.

The reasons for having these designated "workout towels" as part of your equipment are:

1. Safety
2. Hygiene
3. Convenience

Safety is always a matter of concern when working with your dumbbells. If you tend to perspire a lot, you'll want to make sure your hands are dry before you pick up the dumbbell. Also, you'll want to remove moisture from your hands while you're using them so they don't slip. This is an important safety factor. Dumbbells are serious pieces of equipment. Keeping your hands free from moisture will help prevent them from slipping or dropping out of your hands.

Maintaining clean equipment and a safe exercise space is also important. Hygiene and gym etiquette are especially important if you are training where a lot of other people train. Even if your workout area is yours exclusively, it is always a good idea to protect your exercise mat or workbench with a towel.

And as for convenience, that's the premise of this entire chapter! One way to ensure convenience and thus compliance is having your exercise space ready to go when you are. Again, if there is any deterrent, even one as seemingly insignificant as locating a towel, it can get in the way of your energy flow. And once that flow is interrupted, even by minor distractions—having to move, locate equipment, or answer a phone call—you may find it hard to regroup your energy and get on with your workout.

STEP STOOL

I know it doesn't seem like gym equipment, but it is. And I am talking about your basic kitchen-style step stool, the type you pull over to the cabinet when you want to retrieve that hard-to-reach item on the top shelf (well, I do).

A step stool comes in very handy for performing a full range of motion exercises for the feet and ankles, especially an important exercise called heel raises. Heel raises strengthen the backs of the legs and ankle joints and are executed by lifting your heels off the ground and lowering them again. As you become stronger, the advantage to executing this move using a step stool is that you get a much wider range of motion than doing them flat on the floor.

A step stool is also good to use for the more aggressive forms of forward lunges, again by allowing you to move deeper and thus getting a fuller range of motion while working the hip flexors.

As I said, this is an ordinary kitchen step stool that morphs into a valuable piece of gym equipment when used imaginatively (and, of course, safely!). Step stools are very inexpensive, ranging from ten dollars for molded plastic to probably no more than twenty dollars for one that is two-tiered, of metal construction, with slip-resistant material covering the step surfaces. In my gym, I use the ten-dollar plastic stool and it works beautifully.

Your dumbbells, mat, mirror, towels, and step stool are the basics. And as we've calculated so far, the price tag to set you up is less than one hundred dollars!

· extra stuff that's fun to have ·

These are some additional, nonessential items that you may want to consider including at some point:

1. Weight-lifting gloves
2. Dumbbell rack

3. Workout bench
4. Tubes, bands, and balls

WEIGHT-LIFTING GLOVES

One good reason to buy a good, well-fitted pair of gloves is obvious—they protect your hands. Another good reason is they might help you grip the dumbbells better. Nonetheless, some people like them and some people don't. Neoprene dumbbells are covered in vinyl and aren't rough on the hands. But some chrome and iron dumbbells have little ridges on the shafts to help the hands grip better and those may feel uncomfortable. Gloves range in price from thirteen to thirty dollars. Again, it's a personal choice.

DUMBBELL RACK

You can also purchase a dumbbell rack to hold your dumbbells. In fact, often sports equipment and gym equipment stores sell a complete package: dumbbells and a rack to hold them. These sets usually contain three sets of dumbbells. If the sizes are right for you, then a prepackaged set of dumbbell equipment is ideal. They usually range from thirty to sixty dollars.

WORKOUT BENCH

If you have enough space and a flexible budget, I also recommend adding a workout bench at some point. This is not a necessity, by any means. But it is a nice piece of optional equipment that can enhance your dumbbell workouts by helping you maintain the integrity of your form and increase the variety of the exercises you can perform.

If you are seriously considering a bench, I highly recommend one that converts from a flat (horizontal) position to an incline (above horizontal) or decline (below horizontal) position. This type of bench, depending on the manufacturer and additional equipment that can sometimes be added, ranges from around $150 to $300. It is a pricey item but one that may be worth it as your fitness level improves and you become more experienced and confident using your dumbbells.

TUBES, BANDS, AND BALLS

No, this is not the name of a rock group. Tubes, bands, and balls are all resistance mechanisms that can be used in addition to your dumbbells to stimulate muscles and add variety and fun to your workout. All of these items originated in physical therapy and clinical rehabilitative settings. They were used primarily by physical therapists working with people who had suffered orthopedic or neurological damage to help them recover muscle strength, balance, and coordination.

Over the last decade or so, tubes, bands, and balls have migrated out of the clinical setting. They are now commonly used by fitness educators as adjunctive resistance mechanisms in healthy populations in commercial gyms and specifically designed fitness center classes.

Tubes, bands, and balls are usually easily mastered and fairly safe to use. As with all exercise equipment, it is very important to learn how to use them properly to achieve the results you desire without risking injury.

Tubes

Tubes look sort of like jump ropes, but they are actually made of surgical tubing. They come in a wide range of resistance strengths—from extra light to extra heavy—so they are suitable for all fitness levels and needs. You can buy them unadorned, simply the tubes themselves, and now they come with handles or loops to make them easier to grip. There are also specially designed tubes to work specific body parts, like your legs or chest.

The strengths are usually color-keyed to the intensity of their resistance.

YELLOW   Extra light
GREEN   Light
RED   Medium

| BLUE | Heavy |
| BLACK | Extra heavy |

Tubes can provide some modest resistance to work muscles in the arms (biceps and triceps), chest, shoulders, and even a little bit in the legs.

Tubes are also ideal for providing light resistance and facilitating range of motion during stretching.

Additionally, tubes are convenient. You can take them anywhere: your car, a suitcase, even your purse, because they are small and flexible and lightweight. I often make gifts of either tubes or bands. Many of my clients have rigorous travel schedules and want to do some workouts while they're away, but no one seems particularly enthusiastic about packing a set of five-pound dumbbells to haul around on the road.

Flat Bands

Flat bands are used in similar ways to tubes for providing controlled resistance, muscle stimulation, and increased flexibility. They are great mechanisms for intensifying stretches and facilitating range-of-motion activities.

They also come in a wide range of resistance strengths from extra light to extra heavy. Flat bands are also ideal for augmenting stretch reflexes.

Choosing flat bands over the surgical tubing should be based on how you will be working with them—which is easier for you to handle and feels the most comfortable. You want to be able to exercise with control to protect your form and get the results you want, so it is important to feel confident while using them.

Balls

Balls, commonly referred to as Swiss, physio, or exercise balls, have become such a popular and effective device with exercisers these days entire classes are designed around their use. The draw with physio balls is they promote core strengthening, help protect the spine during exercises, increase balance, and promote coordination. Another bonus is they add variety and fun to your workout routine.

Balls are a great tool for working with your dumbbells. You can use the ball in lieu of a bench or chair to perform your upper body dumbbell exercises, lower body squats, and abdominal exercises, as well as a variety of dynamic stretches. The advantage to sitting on an exercise ball when you lift your dumbbells is that it forces you to use your trunk muscles (abs and back) for stability and core strengthening so you don't fall off the ball.

Allover body strength begins with a strong and stable core. A paper published in *ACSM's Health and Fitness Journal* concluded, "Core strength and endurance are paramount to having good core stability and a healthy spine."

One study using electromyography—a test that measures muscle response to nervous stimulation (electrical activity within muscle fibers)—showed that the first muscle groups to activate are the back and abdominal muscles regardless of what other body part a person is working out. In people who suffer from low back problems, however, the first muscle group recruited is the muscle group being trained. What this means is that if you have a strong core, strong abs, and strong erector spinae muscles (back muscles), when you do a biceps curl, the first muscles you recruit are your back and abs for stabilization, even though you aren't working these muscle groups directly!

Exercise balls range from around twenty-five dollars to as much as sixty dollars. Price is based on the quality and size of the ball. The size of the ball that is correct for you is based on your height.

YOUR HEIGHT	APPROPRIATE BALL SIZE
5' to 5'7"	55 cm
5'7" to 6'2"	65 cm

Again, exercise balls are a fabulous addition to your home gym because they are effective, versatile, and fun. Also, they're inexpensive and don't take up too much space.

Remember that you're not only building your home gym, you are building a strategy for a lifetime of health and fitness. This is just the beginning.

You may join a commercial gym or fitness center, but you'll always have the convenience of your own gym available to tide you over during the times when your schedule is less flexible and your exercise time limited. You're not only building your physical strength, you're creating a backup system (sort of like a floppy disc) ensuring your continuation in the Exercise Success Triad.

the smart girls dumbbell exercise recipes and the "30 days and you're on your way" exercise menu

remember in chapter 4 when I explained there are no quick weight loss and exercise fixes? That building a beautiful and healthy body takes time, commitment, and knowledge? Well, I am telling you the truth. That's why I call all the exercise instructions *recipes* . . . because each step is crucial to the desired outcome: creating beautiful muscle. And for equally sound reasons I call my program *30 Days and You're on Your Way*. Not *30 Days and Okay You're Finished*. Or *30 Days and You've Got the Body You've Always Dreamed of and Now You Can Forget about It*.

Because you can't . . . and you won't (not if I've done my job properly).

My goal for you is that through an understanding of the Exercise Success Triad, all the step-by-step exercise (and stretch) recipes, the exercise management tools, and the "30 Days" exercise menu, you'll have the skills and motivation needed to launch you on a lifelong practice of fitness and health. Maybe I should have titled this book *Smart Girls Do Dumbbells for Life*, because it *is* for life and *quality of life* throughout the aging process.

I know some of you are in your twenties or early thirties, and your concerns right now are not focused totally on health but also on the beauty benefits of building muscle and having strong, sexy, attractive bodies. There's absolutely no crime in desiring that! A beautiful physical appearance is a driving force for all of us.

As for those among you who are in your forties and fifties, you are probably wanting the same beauty benefits, but are also seeking to protect your health because you realize that you are losing muscle tone, your formerly fiery metabolism is slowing down, and your energy level is being compromised. You might also be facing some metabolic problems, such as high blood pressure, high blood fat, diabetes, or bone loss. Some of you are in "body shock." Perhaps there's a bit of gravity-based alteration going on and subtle, never-before-experienced expansions.

Our bodies change, dear readers, yes, they do. But Smart Girls—Smart Girls who do dumbbells—*their* bodies change for the best, and for the *best of life*!

· five functional facts to get you started and to keep you going ·

NOW, AN IMPORTANT WORD ABOUT SAFETY

Dumbbells are benign creatures, for the most part. They don't make a lot of noise and are really user-friendly. However, they are heavy, even fairly light ones, and must be handled with care and respect. Below are some general safety guidelines to keep in mind:

- Keep dumbbells away from the delicate hands and feet of small children.

- Never leave dumbbells unattended on a chair or bench where they can roll off and break something valuable, like a Tiffany bowl or your foot.
- Wear shoes or protective footwear when you are working out.
- If you tend to perspire, dry your hands before using dumbbells or wear weight-lifting gloves so they can't slip from your grip.
- Don't leave dumbbells out where someone can trip over them.

SELECTING THE APPROPRIATE-SIZED DUMBBELLS

Start low, go slow
Start low, go slow
Start low, go slow.

That's a motto I'd like to emblazon on all gym walls, fitness facilities, exercise clubs, weight rooms, and anywhere people train with dumbbells. *Start low, go slow!*—I simply can't stress it enough. I have found people are in disbelief when I suggest they start with one- or two-pound dumbbells.

Judy is a perfect example.

"What! Two pounds? What good will *that* do?" she exclaimed during her first training session with me. She was forty-seven years old and had never lifted a dumbbell in her life. "I want muscle but I don't think I'll get much of it with those tiny things."

By the time she got to her third set of ten reps with the two-pounders, she had answered her own question. She had stressed her unused muscles to the max. She was tired, she had worked hard (and with *perfect* form), and, most importantly, she didn't hurt or injure herself in the process. Within three weeks she was using three-pound dumbbells and, shortly thereafter, five-pounders.

If I had started her with a higher weight, it is possible she would have stopped her dumbbell regimen after the first session. If you start with a weight that is too heavy for your fitness and skill level you run the risk of suffering from Over-Training Syndrome (OTS).

Here are the signs and symptoms of OTS:

- Possible injury
- Inappropriate muscle soreness
- Possible lower back, joint, or neck pain
- Anger or frustration, which could lead to termination
- Depression and lack of energy

Additionally, by starting low, Judy experienced her amazing progress in a safe and appropriate manner as her strength increased and she moved up to the next-size dumbbell. She impressed herself with her own gains!

Motto number two: *Never sacrifice form for mass.* This is as important as *Start low, go slow.* If you are lifting a dumbbell beyond your physiological capability, your form will suffer, your body will rebel, you won't be getting the results you desire, and, worst of all, you risk getting an injury.

COUNTING REPETITIONS AND SETS

Each exercise recipe includes the number of repetitions (reps) and sets you will be doing based on your fitness level. A rep is one performance of one exercise—such as lifting the dumbbell and returning it to the starting position. A set is the number of repetitions you perform in a row before resting. A typical set may contain, for example, twelve reps. Depending on your goals and fitness level, you may do a single set of an exercise or multiple sets.

WORKING MUSCLES IN BOTH DIRECTIONS

There are two types of actions in muscle movement—a shortening of the fibers and a lengthening. The shortening action is when your muscle contracts as it works against gravity or resistance. The lengthening action is when your muscle tension resists against the downward pull of gravity or resistance.

It is important to think about both actions when you use your dumbbells. You want to work slowly and make certain you are controlling the movement of the weights during both the lifting (shortening) phase and the releasing (lengthening) phase.

INCREASING THE WEIGHTS

How do you know when to increase the weight?

You increase your weights when you can finish the last three reps of your last set *easily*. Use the "Feelings of Energy Expended" Scale in the appendix to self-evaluate. Also, you can test yourself by asking yourself the following questions:

- Did I complete this set too easily?
- Am I feeling I need to be more challenged?
- Am I physically ready to increase the weight without sacrificing my form or risking injury?

If the answer to these questions is yes, then it's time to move up to the next-size weight.

TESTING THE WATERS

A good way to move up slowly and safely to a higher weight dumbbell is to do what I call "testing the waters." For instance, if you've answered yes to all the questions above, if you used the "Feelings of Energy Expended" Scale and are ready to move up from, say, three-pounders to fives, do your first set of the exercise using the heavier dumbbell, the fives. If you can barely do the last three reps of the first set, in the next set go back to the three to finish the set. During your next training session, once again begin with the fives and see if you can finish two sets this time. Always finish all the reps in each set, even if you have to go down to the lower weight midway through the set.

If you have never lifted dumbbells, start at the Beginner level I give for each exercise recipe. Increase the size of the dumbbells before you move up to the next level. Again, you will know when to move up to the more advanced level if you can complete your set and repetitions easily.

I want to remind you again of one very important point, the third motto: *You are your own best coach!* This is true if you are working with a trainer or working on your own. Nobody knows your body as intimately as you do. Trust yourself and trust your instincts and you can't go wrong. And remember:

1. *Start low, go slow!*
2. *Never sacrifice form for mass!*
3. *You are your own best coach!*

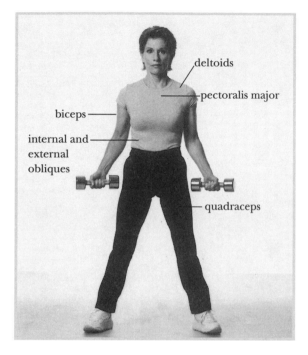

deltoids

pectoralis major

biceps

internal and
external
obliques

quadraceps

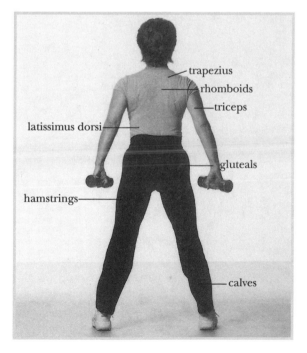

trapezius

rhomboids

triceps

latissimus dorsi

gluteals

hamstrings

calves

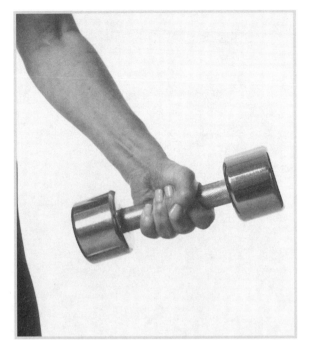

right way
to hold a
dumbbell

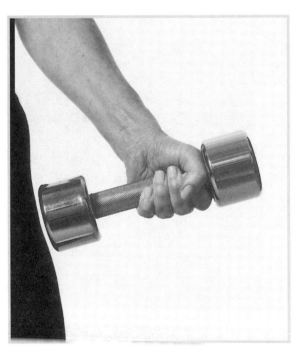

wrong way
to hold a
dumbbell

the
dumbbell exercise
recipes

one-arm overhead extensions

target: back of arms (triceps)

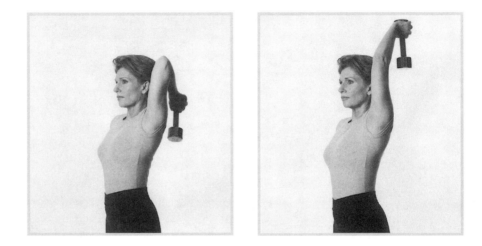

Do One-Arm Overhead Extensions either seated or standing.

FORM

- If standing, place feet shoulder-width apart.
- If seated, sit up straight.
- Keep abdominals contracted throughout the entire exercise.
- Exhale on the extension. Inhale as you lower the dumbbell.
- *Caution: Do not bring the dumbbell too close to your head!*

TECHNIQUE:

- Hold the dumbbell in one hand grasping it by the head, not the shaft.

- Raise your arm so your elbow is as close as possible to the side of your head, near your ear.
- Do not move your arm from this position.
- Extending only your elbow, bring the dumbbell straight up behind and above your head.
- Lower the dumbbell back behind your head as far as possible so you feel the stretch as you lower the dumbbell to the starting position.
- Both the extension and the release should be done slowly and carefully.

· sets and reps ·		
BEGINNER	1 set	10 reps
INTERMEDIATE	2 to 3 scts	10 to 12 reps
ADVANCED	3 sets	12 to 15 reps

exercise recipe #1

exercise recipe #2

two-arm overhead extensions

target: back of arms (triceps)

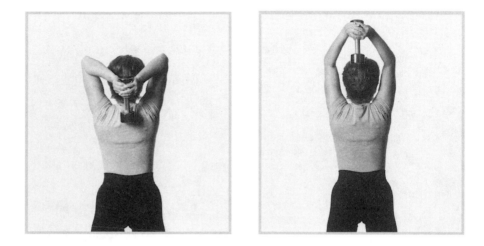

You can do Two-Arm Overhead Extensions either seated or standing.

FORM

- If standing, place feet shoulder-width apart.
- If seated, sit up straight.
- Keep abdominals contracted throughout the entire exercise.
- Exhale on the extension. Inhale as you lower the dumbbell.
- *Caution: Do not bring the dumbbell too close to your head!*

TECHNIQUE

• Hold one dumbbell firmly between both your hands, evenly balanced and grasping it by one head of the dumbbell, not by the shaft. The dumbbell should be level with the back of your head.

• Bring your arms up so your elbows are alongside your head and the dumbbell is not touching the back of your head.

• Extending only your elbows, bring the dumbbell straight up and above your head. (Remember, do not hit yourself in the head. It hurts.)

• Feel a stretch behind your arms, and maybe even underneath your axillary joints (armpits!).

• Lower the dumbbell behind your head as far as possible to the beginning position and you will feel the stretch as you release the dumbbell down.

• Both the extension and the release should be done slowly and carefully.

· sets and reps ·

BEGINNER	1 set	10 reps
INTERMEDIATE	2 to 3 sets	10 to 12 reps
ADVANCED	3 sets	12 to 15 reps

exercise recipe #2

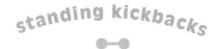

standing kickbacks

target: back of arms (triceps)

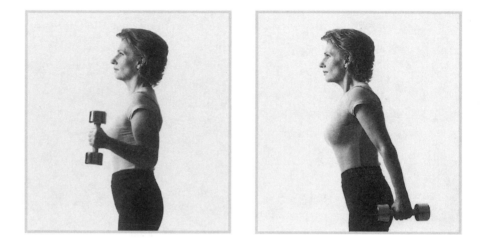

Standing Kickbacks are done one arm at a time.

FORM

- Stand with feet shoulder-width apart and firmly planted to protect your lower back.
- Knees are slight bent.
- Keep abdominals contracted throughout the entire exercise. Very important!
- Exhale on the extension. Inhale as you lower the dumbbell.

TECHNIQUE

- Firmly hold the dumbbell in your hand, evenly balanced.
- Glue the inside of the working arm to the side of your body (rib area). The dumbbell should be aligned with your body.
- As you straighten your elbow by pulling the dumbbell behind you, feel a little squeeze in the triceps muscle.
- Without stopping the flow of the movement, bring the dumbbell back to the starting position.
- Both the extension and the release should be done slowly and carefully.

·sets and reps ·		
BEGINNER	1 set	10 reps
INTERMEDIATE	2 to 3 sets	10 to 12 reps
ADVANCED	3 sets	12 to 15 reps

exercise recipe #3

bent-over kickbacks

target: back of arms (triceps)

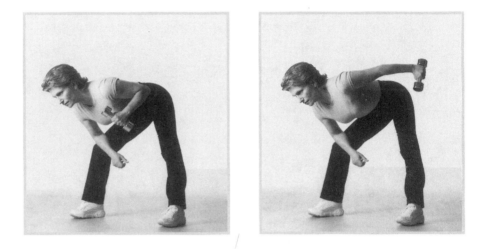

This triceps exercise is done one arm at a time.

FORM

- Begin by placing the foot on the nonworking side of your body about twelve inches in front of you.
- Lean forward and rest the nonworking arm across the top of your extended bent leg. Rest it comfortably, holding no tension in your neck area.
- Contract your abdominals and keep them contracted throughout the entire exercise.
- *Note:* It is especially important to maintain your contraction in this bent-over posture to protect your lower back and prevent the spine from twisting.

TECHNIQUE

- Firmly hold the dumbbell in your free hand (the one *not* placed on your front leg), so that it is aligned with the side of your chest.
- Glue the upper inside of the working arm to the side of your body (rib area) and keep it there without releasing it. Extend your arm back behind you, until your elbow is completely straight.
- Feel a little squeeze in the triceps muscle as you pull the dumbbell back.
- Without stopping the flow of the movement, bring the dumbbell back to the starting position. It should return just about to the side of the breast.
- Both the extension and the release should be done slowly and carefully.

· sets and reps (per arm) ·		
BEGINNER	1 set	10 reps
INTERMEDIATE	2 to 3 sets	10 to 12 reps
ADVANCED	3 sets	12 to 15 reps

exercise recipe #4

v-backs

target: back of arms (triceps)

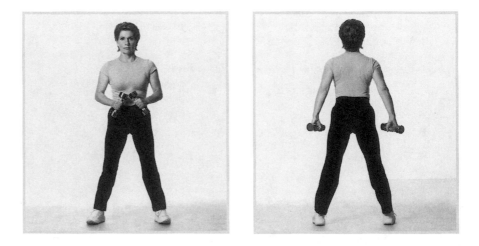

V-Backs can be done either seated or standing.

FORM

* If standing, place feet shoulder-width apart.
* If seated, sit straight, maintaining posture with integrity through-out the entire set.
* Contract your abdominals and keep them contracted throughout the entire exercise.

TECHNIQUE

* Firmly hold the dumbbells in your hands under your breasts and with your elbows sticking out slightly.

- Glue the insides of your upper arms against your rib cage.
- At the same time, extend both hands behind you.
- Keep the triceps muscles contracted as you slowly move your arms behind your back to full extension (no bend in the elbow) as if forming a "V" with your hands.
- Without stopping the flow of movement, bring the dumbbells back to the starting position.
- Both the extension and the release should be done slowly.

· sets and reps ·		
BEGINNER	1 set	10 reps
INTERMEDIATE	2 to 3 sets	10 to 12 reps
ADVANCED	3 scts	12 to 15 reps

exercise recipe #5

classic forward curls

target: front of arms (biceps)

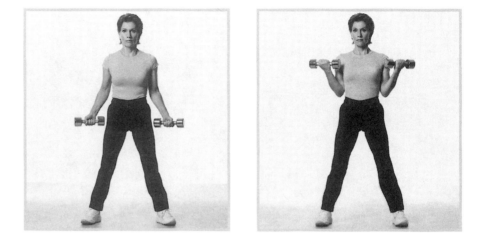

Classic Forward Curls target both the short head and the long head of the biceps, the muscles on the front of your upper arms.

FORM

• Stand facing a mirror, if possible, placing feet shoulder-width apart.
• Plant feet firmly on the ground to keep spine and back stable.
• Contract your abdominals and hold the contraction throughout the entire exercise.
• Relax your neck, shoulders, and head. The only muscles working are the biceps.

TECHNIQUE

- Hold the dumbbells firmly so they remain stable in your hands, but not so tightly that you are squeezing them.
- They should be equally balanced in the palms of your hands.
- The dumbbells are at the sides of your thighs, and your fingers are wrapped around the dumbbells, so you can see your fingertips.
- Slowly bring the dumbbells up using a count to six. Feel the biceps muscles squeeze (contract) as you curl up.
- Using the same count of six, lower the dumbbells to the starting position. Feel the muscles lengthen against the pull of gravity.
- Do not stop between reps but move the dumbbells with a continuous flowing action.
- On these curls you exhale as you bring the dumbbells up toward your shoulders and inhale as you lower them.

· sets and reps ·		
BEGINNER	1 set	10 reps
INTERMEDIATE	2 to 3 sets	10 to 12 reps
ADVANCED	3 sets	12 to 15 reps

exercise recipe #6

supinated curls

target: front of arms (biceps)

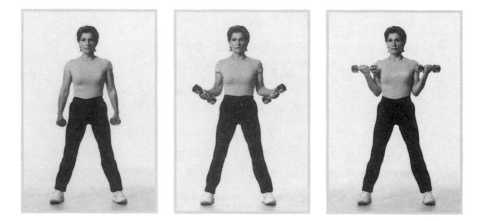

Supinated Curls engage the muscles that twist the wrists, and allow you to work first the front and then the side of the biceps as you turn your wrist.

FORM

- Place feet shoulder-width apart.
- Plant feet firmly on the ground to keep spine and back stable.
- Contract your abdominals and keep them contracted throughout the entire exercise.
- Relax your neck, shoulders, and head. Focus on the biceps muscles as you do the curl.

TECHNIQUE

- Hold the dumbbells firmly, but do not squeeze them so hard that you are expending all your energy holding them.

- They should be equally balanced in your hands.
- Slowly bring the dumbbells up. As you do, turn them so you can see your fingertips coming toward your shoulders. Your elbows should be close by your sides.
- As you return the dumbbells to the starting position, slowly reverse the movements, turning the wrists so fingertips end up once again facing the sides of the legs.
- Remember to move the dumbbells slowly and continuously, feeling both the contraction and the extension of the muscles.
- Exhale as you bring the dumbbells up toward your shoulders and inhale as you lower them.

· sets and reps ·		
BEGINNER	1 set	10 reps
INTERMEDIATE	2 to 3 sets	10 to 12 reps
ADVANCED	3 sets	12 to 15 reps

exercise recipe #7

hammer curls

target: front of arms (biceps)

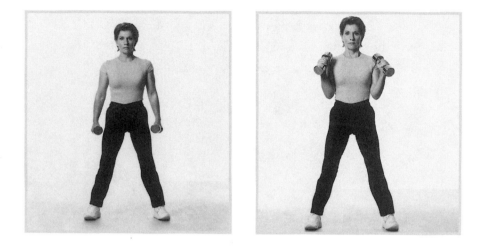

FORM

- Stand with feet shoulder-width apart.
- Plant feet firmly on the ground to keep spine and back stable.
- Contract your abdominals and keep them contracted throughout the entire exercise.
- Relax your neck, shoulders, and head. Focus on the biceps muscles as you do the curl.

TECHNIQUE

- Hold the dumbbells firmly, equally balanced in your hands.
- Start with your arms hanging down by your sides and your fingertips facing toward the sides of your thighs.

- Slowly bring the dumbbells up, leading with their heads and moving in the direction of your shoulders.
- Return to the starting position with the other head of the dumbbell. Remember to move the dumbbells slowly and continuously, feeling both the contraction and the lengthening of the muscles.
- Exhale as you bring the dumbbells up toward your shoulders and inhale as you lower them.

· sets and reps ·		
BEGINNER	1 set	10 reps
INTERMEDIATE	2 to 3 sets	10 to 12 reps
ADVANCED	3 sets	12 to 15 reps

exercise recipe #8

seated one-arm biceps curls

target: front of arms (biceps)

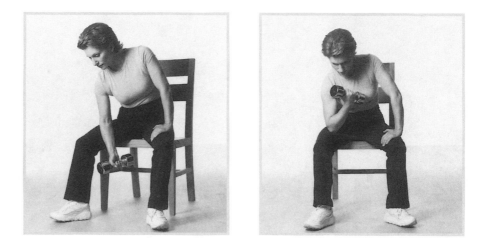

If you want to seriously work your biceps, Seated One-Arm Biceps Curls will increase your level of intensity. They double the time it takes to complete your sets but if you really want that extra concentration, they are the best exercise to do.

FORM

- These biceps curls are done seated and, of course, one arm at a time!
- Sitting on a firm bench or chair, plant feet firmly on the ground.
- Place feet far enough apart so you can lean forward and rest the elbow of the working arm inside the inner thigh, closer to the knee than the upper thigh.
- Relax your neck, shoulders, and head. The only muscles working are the biceps.

TECHNIQUE

- Hold the dumbbell firmly with a good grip.
- Slowly curl the dumbbell toward your shoulder using full range of motion, concentrating on both the contraction (upward motion) and the lengthening (downward motion).
- With equal speed, release the dumbbell to the starting position and as you do, feel the muscles lengthening.
- Do not stop between reps, but move the dumbbell with a continuous flowing action.
- Exhale on the effort (upward motion) and inhale on the release (downward motion).

· sets and reps (per arm) ·		
BEGINNER	1 set	10 reps
INTERMEDIATE	2 to 3 sets	10 to 12 reps
ADVANCED	3 sets	12 to 15 reps

exercise recipe #9

combination biceps curls

target: front of arms (biceps)

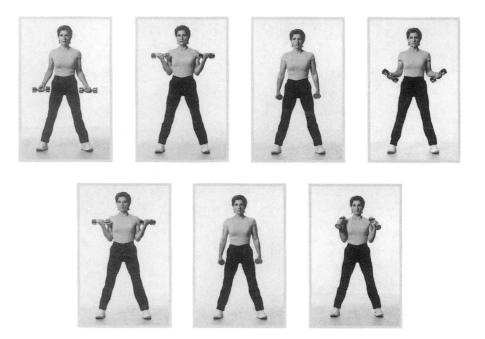

In one set, you can combine Classic Forward, Supinated, and Hammer Curls by doing one exercise followed by the next to complete the set. This adds great variety to your arm set. You can do them seated or standing. I prefer standing to help build core strength but seated is fine if you have a bad lower back, feel insecure about your form, or just prefer being seated while using dumbbells.

FORM

· If you are standing, place feet firmly on the ground, shoulder-width apart. Contract your abs.

- If seated, sit on a firm chair or bench. It should be comfortable, but avoid a chair with a soft cushion seat. Do not do curls on sofas, club chairs, or any chair that does not provide good support.
- Even if you are seated, keep the abdominal muscles contracted to protect the back.

TECHNIQUE

- Hold the dumbbells firmly with a good grip.
- Always use full range of motion, concentrating on both the contraction (upward motion) and the lengthening (downward motion).
- Do not rush the movements. Move the dumbbells slowly in each exercise, with equal speed, generally to a count of six, on both the contraction (upward motion) and the release (downward motion).
- Exhale on the effort (upward motion) and inhale on the release.

· sets and reps ·		
BEGINNER	1 set	3 Classic Forward, 3 Supinated, 3 Hammer Curls
INTERMEDIATE	3 sets	10 Classic Forward, 10 Supinated, 10 Hammer Curls
ADVANCED	3 sets	12 Classic Forward, 12 Supinated, 12 Hammer Curls

exercise recipe #10

exercise recipe #11

side lateral raises

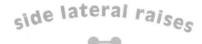

target: top of shoulders

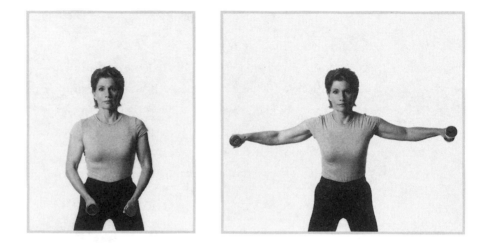

The shoulder muscle is called the deltoid. It is a three-dimensional muscle with fibers on the top, back, and front of the shoulder. This exercise is excellent for strengthening the entire shoulder muscle.

FORM

- If standing, place feet shoulder-width apart to create a solid base.
- If seated, sit up straight.
- Keep abdominals contracted throughout the entire exercise whether you are standing or seated.
- *Please keep a slight bend in your elbows.*

TECHNIQUE

- Firmly hold the dumbbells in your hands, evenly balanced.
- In the starting position, your arms hang in front of your pelvic bone.
- Slowly extend your arms out to the sides, as if taking position to fly. The dumbbells should end up level with your shoulders.
- Return with equal speed and control to the starting position.
- Do not stop the action when you return to the starting position. Moves should flow evenly up and down.

· sets and reps ·		
BEGINNER	1 set	10 reps
INTERMEDIATE	2 to 3 sets	10 to 12 reps
ADVANCED	3 sets	12 to 15 reps

exercise recipe #11

military presses

target: top of shoulders (deltoids)

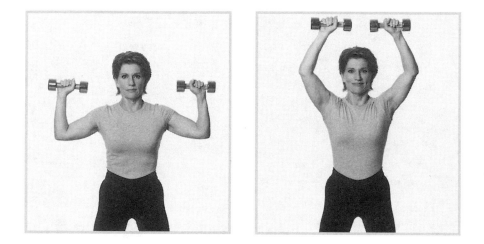

This exercise also focuses on strengthening the entire shoulder muscle—top, back, and front.

FORM

- Place feet shoulder-width apart to create a solid base.
- If seated, sit up straight; do not let your back rest on the chair or bench.
- Keep abdominals contracted throughout the entire exercise, whether you are standing or seated.
- As you perform the exercise, try not to bring the dumbbells too far in front of you or too far behind, just as if they were extensions of your shoulders themselves.

TECHNIQUE

- Starting position: Firmly hold the dumbbells in your hands, keeping the wrists steady and the dumbbells evenly balanced. Your elbows should be bent and the dumbbells held slightly above your shoulders.
- Raise the dumbbells up slowly, lifting them above the top of your head. The dumbbells move together as they rise above your head until they are almost touching at the top.
- In one fluid motion, bring the dumbbells back down to the starting position at the sides of the shoulders.
- Remember to *control the downward motion* as you return the dumbbells to the starting position—so you are working the muscles during both the lifting and the downward phase.

· sets and reps ·		
BEGINNER	1 set	10 reps
INTERMEDIATE	2 to 3 sets	10 to 12 reps
ADVANCED	3 sets	12 to 15 reps

exercise recipe #12

upright rows

●━●

target: front of shoulders (anterior deltoids)

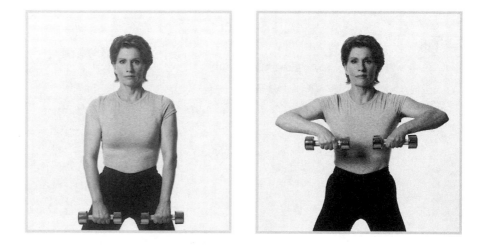

There is a little muscle in the front of the shoulder called the anterior
(front) deltoid. The Upright Row exercise targets this front shoulder muscle specifically. It is important to work on this muscle because it helps stabilize the shoulder joint for racket sports, swimming, and golf, plus it
makes your shoulders look great in strapless dresses.

FORM

* If you are doing this exercise standing, place feet shoulder-width
apart to create your solid working base.
* If seated, sit up straight; do not let your back rest on the chair or
bench back.
* Keep abdominals contracted throughout the entire exercise,
whether standing or seated.

TECHNIQUE

- Starting position: Firmly hold the dumbbells in your hands. The dumbbells are hanging in front of your thighs, wrists turned inward so your fingers are facing toward your body.
- Raise the dumbbells up toward your shoulders. As you bring them up, your elbows go out to the sides. (It is the same motion as if you were pulling your panty hose up over your head.)
- Return the dumbbells to the starting position in front of the top of the thighs.
- Remember to keep the movements flowing and don't stop either at the starting or the ending position.

· sets and reps ·

BEGINNER	1 set	10 reps
INTERMEDIATE	2 to 3 sets	10 to 12 reps
ADVANCED	3 sets	12 to 15 reps

exercise recipe #13

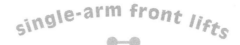

single-arm front lifts

target: front of shoulders (anterior deltoids)

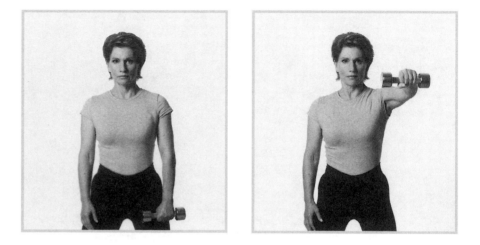

Single-Arm Front Lifts also work the front shoulder muscle, but they are a little more difficult, and form is very important. You may have to use a lighter dumbbell than you use in the Upright Rows because of the increased difficulty.

FORM

- If you are doing this exercise standing, place feet shoulder-width apart to create your solid working base.
- If seated, sit up straight; do not let your back rest on the chair or bench back.
- Keep abdominals contracted throughout the entire exercise, whether you are standing or seated.
- This is very important: Keep a slight bend in your elbow to prevent injury to the joint.

• It is best to do this exercise one arm at a time, alternating left and right, to protect your form.

TECHNIQUE

• Starting position: Firmly hold the dumbbell in your hand. The dumbbell is hanging in front of your thigh, wrists turned inward so your fingertips are facing toward your leg. There is a very slight flexion in the wrists with fingertips facing toward the ground.
• Lift the dumbbell away from your body bringing it straight out in front of you. Remember to keep the elbow slightly bent.
• Continue lifting until the dumbbell is slightly higher than your shoulder.
• Immediately return the dumbbell to the starting position in front of the top of the thigh.
• Repeat with the other arm.

· sets and reps ·		
BEGINNER	1 set	10 reps
INTERMEDIATE	2 to 3 sets	10 to 12 reps
ADVANCED	3 sets	12 to 15 reps

exercise recipe #14

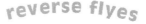

reverse flyes

target: back of shoulders (posterior deltoids)

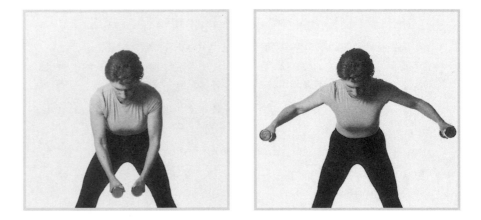

The back of the shoulder muscle is worked by abducting the arm (bringing it away from the body) in a motion that feels like you are squeezing your shoulder blades together. It is the reverse action of traditional flyes (which are a "hugging a beach ball" move).

FORM

- It is best to do this exercise standing to allow for full range of motion, but it can be done seated on the edge of a chair or bench.
- If you are doing this exercise standing, place feet shoulder-width apart to create your solid working base.
- If seated, sit up straight; do not let your back rest on the chair or bench back.
- Keep abdominals contracted throughout the entire exercise, whether standing or seated.
- Keep a slight bend in your elbows to protect the elbow joints.

TECHNIQUE

- Firmly hold the dumbbells evenly balanced in your hands.
- Bend forward slightly at the waist, enough so that your torso is facing toward the floor. Remember, keep those abs especially tight in this position to protect your lower back.
- Start with the dumbbells in front of your legs, but away from the body, hanging loosely in front of you.
- Fingertips are facing one another so the dumbbells are parallel.
- Bring the dumbbells out to your sides, as if you were a bird spreading out your wings. Remember to keep your elbows slightly bent.
- In this position, they come just level with your shoulders.
- You feel the contraction in the rear of your shoulders and some in your upper back.
- Lower the dumbbells to the starting position, controlling the movement and maintaining your form.

· sets and reps ·		
BEGINNER	1 set	10 reps
INTERMEDIATE	2 to 3 sets	10 to 12 reps
ADVANCED	3 sets	12 to 15 reps

exercise recipe #15

bench presses

target: chest (pectoralis major)

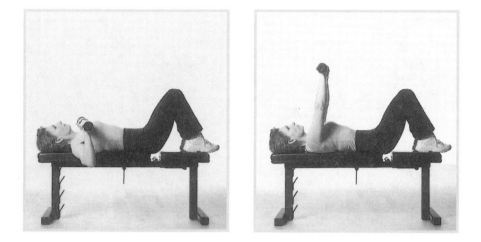

Bench Presses are done in a supine (face upward) position lying on a bench or the floor. The muscle fibers of the chest attach to the humerus (the upper-arm bone) and it is therefore best to do these presses on some sort of bench to allow for full range of motion.

FORM

- Lie on a flat bench (or floor), bend your knees, and place your feet flat on the surface in front of you to protect your lower back.
- Keep abdominals contracted as you lift the dumbbells.

TECHNIQUE

- Start with the dumbbells aligned with your shoulders, slightly above the breasts.

- Bring the dumbbells up, above your chest in a semicircle motion so they come together—but don't slam the dumbbells into each other!
- Squeeze the chest wall as you move the dumbbells toward one another.
- Release dumbbells slowly to the starting position. This downward move is very important! Don't let the dumbbells just drop, but control them all the way down to the starting position. As you lower them, you are working your triceps by controlling the motion.

· sets and reps ·		
BEGINNER	1 set	10 reps
INTERMEDIATE	2 to 3 sets	10 to 12 reps
ADVANCED	3 sets	12 to 15 reps

exercise recipe #16

exercise recipe #17

bench flyes

target: chest (pectoralis major)

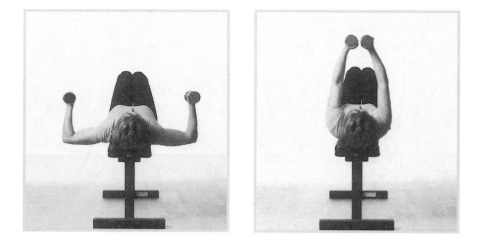

Flyes are the moves that imitate hugging a beach ball or barrel. Do them lying on a bench or the floor, knees bent to protect your lower back.

FORM

• Lying on a flat bench (or floor), hold the dumbbells at shoulder height, with your wrists facing each other.
• Keep abdominals contracted as you lift the dumbbells.
• Keep elbows slightly bent.

TECHNIQUE

• Bring the dumbbells toward one another as if you were hugging a barrel. Bring the dumbbells up above your chest in a semicircle motion, so they come together at the top—but don't slam the dumb-bells into each other.

- Release dumbbells slowly to the starting position. This downward move is very important! Don't let the dumbbells just drop, but control them all the way down to the starting position. As you lower them, you are working your triceps by controlling the motion.

· sets and reps ·		
BEGINNER	1 set	10 reps
INTERMEDIATE	2 to 3 sets	10 to 12 reps
ADVANCED	3 sets	12 to 15 reps

exercise recipe #17

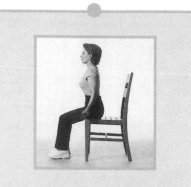

smart girls sit up straight

For exercise recipes #18 and #19 (and for any of the dumbbell exercises you do while seated), posture is very important. It is best to use a chair or bench with a solid seat. Sit at the edge, planting your feet firmly on the ground. Contract your abdominal muscles, sit tall, keep your shoulders relaxed and your chin lifted. This will help protect your lower back and spine, and start retraining your body to sit and stand properly even when not exercising! Try to hold this posture consistently throughout the exercise, and don't let your movements of the dumbbells sacrifice your form. If it feels difficult to lift and stay upright completely, then you may want to reduce the weight in the beginning. And remember: no slouching!

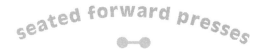

seated forward presses

target: chest (pectoralis major)

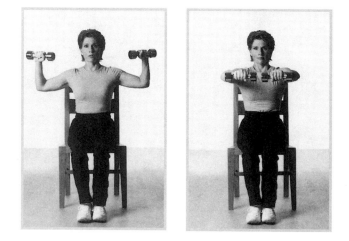

You can do Seated Forward Presses on the edge of a bench or in a chair, as long as your back is not resting on the chair back.

FORM

• Sit up tall, pulling up from your core (your central trunk), abs contracted and spine straight.

• Relax your neck and shoulders. No tension!

• Place feet firmly on the ground hip distance apart.

• Keep abdominals contracted as you lift the dumbbells.

TECHNIQUE

* Start with the dumbbells held by the tops of your shoulders, your wrists facing forward.
* Push the dumbbells forward in front of your chest in a single smooth motion.
* At the farthest reaching point away from your body—while keeping a slight bend in the elbows—move the heads of the dumbbells together.
* Release the dumbbells slowly, controlling them all the way to the starting position by the tops of your shoulders.
* Generally, this should be a smooth, flowing movement that you feel right across the top of the chest.

· sets and reps ·		
BEGINNER	1 set	10 reps
INTERMEDIATE	2 to 3 sets	10 to 12 reps
ADVANCED	3 sets	12 to 15 reps

exercise recipe #18

seated forward flyes

target: chest (pectoralis major)

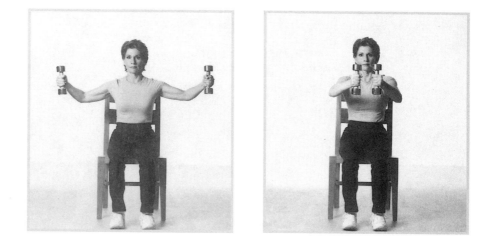

Like the Bench Flyes, the Seated Forward Flyes are a "hugging a beach ball" movement. Do this exercise on the edge of a bench or in a chair (as long as your back is not resting against the chair).

FORM

- Sit up tall, pulling up from your core, abs contracted and spine straight.
- Relax your neck and shoulders.
- Place feet firmly on the ground hip distance apart.
- Keep abdominals contracted.

TECHNIQUE

• Start with the handles of the dumbbells held vertically, with the upper heads even with the tops of your shoulders. Your wrists should be facing one another.

• Curve the dumbbells in front of your chest, keeping your elbows bent, as if you were hugging someone.

• Your arms should be about twenty inches in front of your body and about level with your breasts.

• As you bring the dumbbells in front of you, concentrate on "squeezing" the chest muscles, feeling a flexlike sensation.

• At the farthest reaching point away from your body—while keeping a slight bend in the elbows—move the dumbbells together.

• It should feel as if you are encircling a beach ball between your arms.

• Release the dumbbells slowly to the starting position. Control them all the way to the starting position.

• Generally, this should be a smooth, flowing movement that you feel right across the top of your chest.

· sets and reps ·

BEGINNER	1 set	10 reps
INTERMEDIATE	2 to 3 sets	10 to 12 reps
ADVANCED	3 sets	12 to 15 reps

exercise recipe #19

standing bent-over rows

target: back (trapezius, latissimus dorsi, and rhomboids)

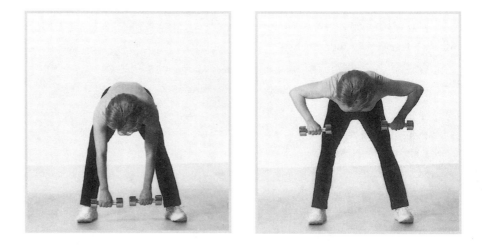

This exercise for back muscles is done standing.

FORM

- You begin by taking one dumbbell in each hand. Slowly bend over forward, so your chest is parallel to the floor.
- Your spine is in a neutral position (do not arch it or sink it) and your abdominal muscles are contracted to protect your lower back.
- Knees are slightly bent.
- Buttocks are squeezed tightly.
- Relax your neck and shoulders, but keep your abs contracted to protect your back throughout the movement.

TECHNIQUE

• Start with your arms hanging down in front of you with your wrists facing toward your body, so the shafts of the dumbbells are parallel to the floor.
• Bring the dumbbells up to your sides by bending your elbows pointing outward.
• Squeeze your shoulder blades together as you lift the dumbbells.
• Exhale as you bring the dumbbells up and inhale as you lower them to the starting position.
• As you release the dumbbells to the starting position, make certain you *control* the downward movement.

· sets and reps ·		
BEGINNER	1 sct	10 reps
INTERMEDIATE	2 to 3 sets	10 to 12 reps
ADVANCED	3 sets	12 to 15 reps

exercise recipe #20

kneeling one-arm rows

target: back (trapezius, latissimus dorsi, and rhomboids)

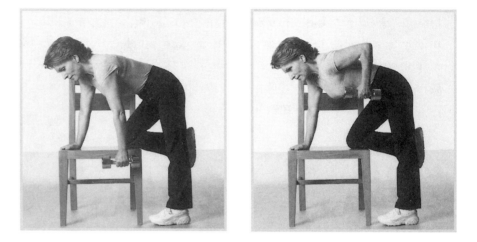

Your back is composed of large muscles, so you can usually lift a little heavier than with smaller muscle groups, like shoulders or triceps. To do this exercise, you will need a bench or chair on which you can lean with a bent knee with room to place your hand in front of you to keep your body aligned.

FORM

- Place one knee on the bench and kneel over, placing your hand in front of you to stabilize your body.
- Relax your neck and shoulders, but keep your abs contracted to protect your back.
- Your spine should be in a neutral position; do not arch the back or sluk into the position.

TECHNIQUE

- The shaft of the dumbbell is in the hand on the side of your body next to the standing leg.
- Starting position: The working arm hangs alongside the standing leg.
- Without allowing the dumbbell to twist or turn in your hand, bring it straight up, alongside your rib cage, squeezing your back muscles as you lift the dumbbell.
- Release the dumbbell to the starting position slowly and with control.

· sets and reps (per arm) ·		
BEGINNER	1 set	10 reps
INTERMEDIATE	2 to 3 sets	10 to 12 reps
ADVANCED	3 sets	12 to 15 reps

exercise recipe #21

front squats

target: front of legs and buttocks
(quadriceps and gluteals)

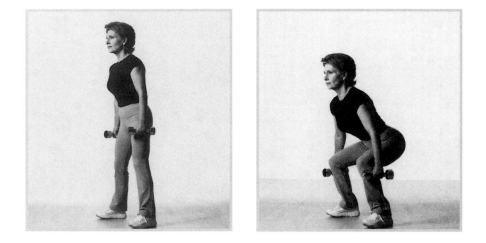

The Front Squat is a multijointed exercise that is accomplished by flexing the knees and flexing the hips. The advantage to doing a multijointed exercise is that you work two muscle groups at once!

FORM

- Place feet hip-width apart.
- Before you start the squat, contract your abs.
- Toes are pointing forward.
- Do not let your knees protrude beyond your toes when you squat.

TECHNIQUE

- Hold the dumbbells either down by the sides of your legs or if you prefer, curled up toward your chest.

- The dumbbells do not move separately, but are used in the squat to provide resistance.
- Bend your knees and lower your buttocks as you would do to sit down in a chair.
- When your thighs are parallel to the ground you have dropped deep enough.
- Make certain your knees are pointed straight ahead but *do not go out over your toes*!
- Squeeze your buttock muscles tightly and keep the abs contracted.
- Make certain your spine is straight, although your trunk may be bent slightly forward.
- Once you've reached the squat position, continue to squeeze your buttocks and contract your abs as you return to standing.
- Squats should be done slowly and with a high degree of concentration.

· sets and reps ·

BEGINNER	1 set	5 to 10 reps
INTERMEDIATE	1 set	10 to 20 reps
ADVANCED	1 set	20 to 30 reps

exercise recipe #22

exercise recipe #23

forward lunges

target: front of legs and buttocks
(quadriceps and gluteals)

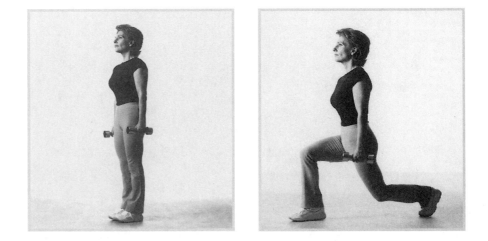

Lunges are another form of multijointed exercise that targets both your quads (front of your legs) and your buttocks. If you have good knees they are one of the best buttocks-tightening exercises you can do. If you have good balance, you can do these without holding on to anything, but if you don't, just place the hand of your nonworking leg on a counter or wall to keep you steady as you do the Forward Lunges.

FORM

- Stand tall, abs contracted.
- If you have only one free hand, hold one dumbbell at your side and keep it steady.
- If both hands are free, hold a dumbbell in each hand at your sides and keep them steady.

- As you lunge forward, make sure your trunk remains tall.
- Do not slouch over as you lunge.

TECHNIQUE

- Place your working leg a long step forward and bend your knee, dropping into a forward lunge.
- The knee of the non-lunging leg drops toward the ground into a ninety-degree angle.
- Make sure your knee *does not come out over your toes*!
- Squeeze your buttock muscles tightly and keep the abs contracted the entire time.
- Make certain your back remains straight and your body does not go out of alignment.
- Hold the lunge position for about three to five seconds, then bring the foot back to its starting position.
- Repeat with the other leg.
- Lunges should be done slowly, with deep concentration, paying special attention to form and execution.

· sets and reps ·

BEGINNER	1 set	5 to 10 reps
INTERMEDIATE	1 set	10 to 20 reps
ADVANCED	1 set	20 to 30 reps

exercise recipe #23

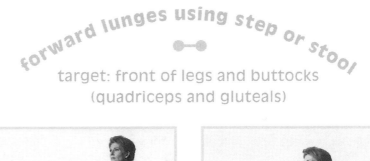

forward lunges using step or stool

target: front of legs and buttocks
(quadriceps and gluteals)

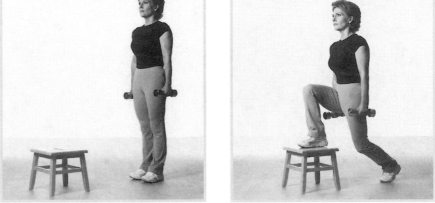

Lunging on a step or stool intensifies the Forward Lunge but you need to have good knees. If you have good balance, you can hold a dumbbell in each hand. If not, or if you feel it is too hard to lunge and balance, hold on to a counter with one hand and place the dumbbell in the hand of the forward-lunging leg.

FORM

- Stand tall, abs contracted.
- Hold the dumbbells at your sides and keep them steady.
- As you lunge forward, make sure your spine is straight.
- Do not bend forward or slouch over as you execute the lunge.

TECHNIQUE

• Bring your working leg forward into a lunge as you place the ball of your foot onto the stair or step.

• Lunge forward, making sure your knee *does not come out over your toes*!

• The knee of the non-lunging leg drops toward the ground into a ninety-degree angle.

• Squeeze your buttock muscles tight and keep the abdominal muscles contracted the entire time.

• Make certain your back is straight, your shoulders squared, and your body in alignment.

• Hold the lunge position for about three to five seconds, then bring the foot back to its starting position.

• Do all your reps using the same leg, then switch to the other leg.

· sets and reps ·

BEGINNER	1 set	5 to 10 reps
INTERMEDIATE	1 set	10 to 20 reps
ADVANCED	1 set	20 to 30 reps

walking lunges

target: front of legs and buttocks
(quadriceps and gluteals)

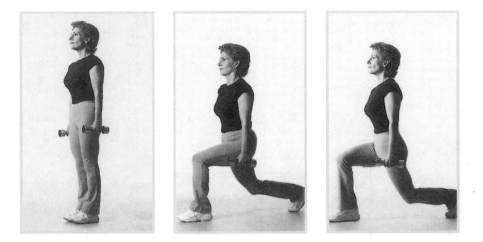

If you have good balance and feel comfortable moving while holding dumbbells, Walking Lunges are a superior exercise to help tighten the buttocks and strengthen the quads. You will need some room in front of you, as the Walking Lunges move you forward, so a hallway or wide room will do.

FORM

- Hold a dumbbell in each hand, wrists facing inward, the dumbbell shafts parallel to the sides of your upper thighs.
- Posture is critical as you lunge forward.
- Keep your abs contracted.
- Your trunk remains tall, back straight, chest open, and head high.

TECHNIQUE

• Lunge forward with each step.

• You are in the ideal lunge position when the thigh of your lunging leg is parallel to the ground and the knee of the rear leg is at a ninety-degree angle.

• Make sure your knee *does not come out over your toes*!

• Squeeze your buttock muscles tight and keep the abs contracted the entire time.

• Make certain your back remains straight and your body does not go out of alignment.

• Hold the lunge position for about three seconds, squeezing the buttocks, then with your other leg take the next lunge step forward.

· sets and reps ·		
BEGINNER	1 set	5 to 10 reps
INTERMEDIATE	2 sets	10 to 15 reps
ADVANCED	3 sets	15 to 20 reps

exercise recipe #25

reverse lunges

target: front of legs and buttocks
(quadriceps and gluteals)

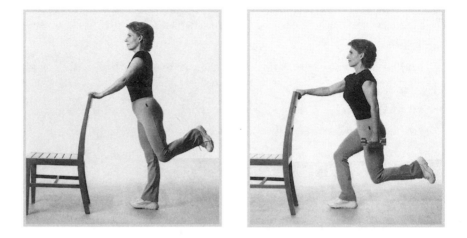

In Reverse Lunges you lunge backward instead of forward. You do these one leg at a time holding on to a ballet bar, the back of a chair, a countertop or any stationary surface.

FORM

- The non-lunging leg is bent behind you at a ninety-degree angle.
- Place a dumbbell in the hand next to the non-lunging leg, wrist facing inward, the dumbbell shaft parallel to the side of your thigh.
- Posture is critical as you lunge backward.
- Keep your abs contracted, trunk tall, back straight, chest open, and head high.

TECHNIQUE

* Holding on to a chair, bar, or countertop, push yourself backward from a standing position, leading with your buttocks as if you were going to sit down in a chair.
* As you lunge backward, drop your bent knee as deeply as you can toward the ground.
* Protect the knee of the lunging leg by making certain it does *not go out over the toes.*
* Squeeze your buttock muscles tightly and keep the abs contracted the entire time as you perform each lunge backward.
* Hold the lunge position for about three seconds and return to standing position.
* After you complete a full set with one leg, switch to the other leg.

· sets and reps ·		
BEGINNER	1 set	5 to 10 reps
INTERMEDIATE	2 sets	10 to 15 reps
ADVANCED	3 sets	15 to 20 reps

exercise recipe #26

deadlifts

target: back of legs (hamstrings) and lower back

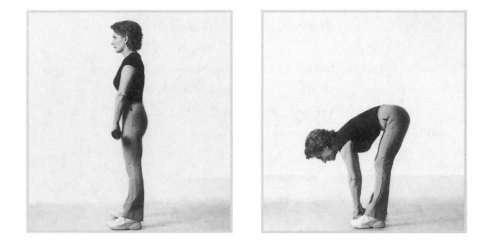

This is the ideal exercise to work the hamstrings and the erector spinae muscle group, which extends on each side of the spinal column. It is best if you can do Deadlifts on a step or a slightly raised platform to get a full range of motion.

FORM

- Hold a dumbbell in each hand.
- Hold your arms slightly out in front of you, wrists facing your thighs with the shafts of the dumbbells parallel to your body.
- Stand with your feet hip distance apart.
- Abs are contracted and spine is straight.

TECHNIQUE

• Carefully bend forward, lowering the dumbbells toward the ground in front of you; drop down as deeply as possible but keep a slight bend in your knees.

• You do not want to lock out or hyperextend the knees, as this can cause problems in your knee joints.

• After you bend over as far as you can, slowly start to come up again.

• Make sure you come up slowly, one vertebra at a time.

• Abs are contracted the entire time!

• Your head is the last thing to come up.

• When you are once again standing upright, move your upper body very slightly backward, squeezing your buttocks together tightly. This is a gentle hyperextension and really focuses on the upper buttocks/lower back area.

· sets and reps ·

BEGINNER	1 set	5 to 10 reps
INTERMEDIATE	2 sets	10 to 15 reps
ADVANCED	3 sets	15 to 20 reps

exercise recipe #27

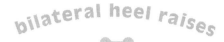

bilateral heel raises

target: calves and ankles

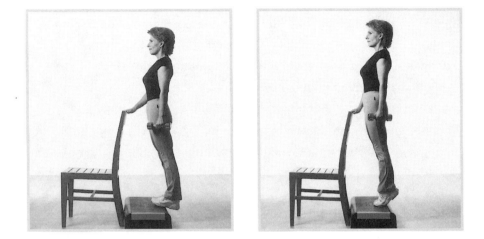

Heel Raises work the two muscles of the calves. They also help strengthen the complex of little bones, muscles, and ligaments in the feet and ankles. Strong feet and ankles help with posture, balance, and overall endurance.

It helps to do these exercises on a step, stair, or step stool to achieve full range of flexion in the feet. You should hold on to a wall, countertop, or the back of a chair for balance.

FORM

* Place both feet on the step or stool.
* Hold a dumbbell in one hand, wrist facing toward the body with the shaft of the dumbbell parallel to your leg.
* Bring your feet to the edge of the step, so the toes are just on the edge.

- Abs remain contracted the entire time.
- Your back is straight, head facing forward, shoulders relaxed.

TECHNIQUE

- With your toes on the edge of the stool, slowly lift your heels up as high as you can.
- You will feel a deep contraction in the upper part of the calf muscles.
- Slowly begin to drop your heels down as deeply as possible, below horizontal.
- You will now feel a stretch more in the lower part of the calves and in the heel cords.
- Keep a slight bend in the knees at all times.
- Do half the reps holding the dumbbell on one side and then switch the dumbbell to the other; use the hand not holding the dumbbell to help you balance if you are on a platform.

· sets and reps ·		
BEGINNER	1 set	10 to 15 reps
INTERMEDIATE	2 sets	15 to 20 reps
ADVANCED	3 sets	20 to 25 reps

exercise recipe #28

unilateral heel raises

target: calves and ankles

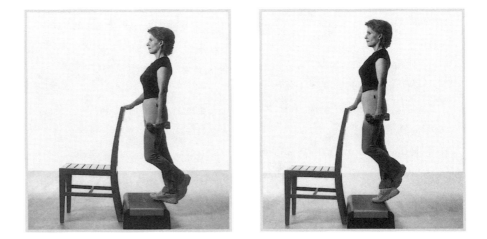

Once again, if you have good balance, it helps to do these Heel Raises on a step, stair, or step stool to achieve full range of flexion in the feet.

FORM

- Stand on the step or stool and wrap one foot around the other's ankle.
- Hold a dumbbell on the side of the working leg (the one supporting your weight), wrist facing toward the body and shaft of the dumbbell parallel to your leg.
- Your toes are just at the edge of the stool or step.
- Abs remain contracted the entire time.
- Your back is straight, head facing forward, shoulders relaxed.

TECHNIQUE

- With your toes on the edge of the stool, slowly lift your heel up as high as you can.
- You will feel a deep contraction in the upper part of the calf muscles.
- When you've lifted your heel as high as you can, slowly begin to drop it down as deeply as possible, below horizontal.
- You will now feel a stretch more in the lower part of the calf and in the heel cord.
- Do half the reps holding the dumbbell on the working-leg side and then switch the dumbbell to the other hand; use your free hand to hold on to the counter, wall, or chair back for balance.

· sets and reps (per leg) ·		
BEGINNER	1 set	10 to 15 reps
INTERMEDIATE	2 sets	15 to 20 reps
ADVANCED	3 sets	20 to 25 reps

exercise recipe #29

plié squats

target: inner thighs (adductors and abductors)

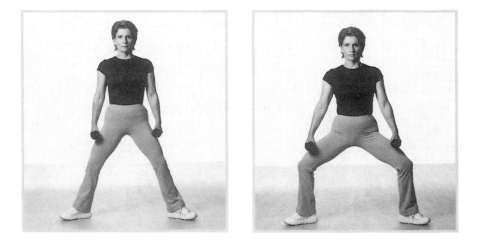

Plié Squats are multijointed exercises that target the inner thigh muscles (adductors) as well as the quads. It is important to maintain good form and technique to protect both the knees and the back while doing Plié Squats.

FORM

- Stand with your feet a little wider than hip-distance apart.
- Toes are pointed outward.
- Contract your abs and hold your spine straight.
- Hold one dumbbell in each hand.
- The shaft of the dumbbells are parallel to the thigh.

TECHNIQUE

- Squat down slowly.
- As you are dropping into the squat, make sure your knees *do not go out over your toes.*
- When you are in the squat position, feel the stretch in your inner thighs.
- Move out of the squat to the upright position by squeezing the muscles of the inner thighs together, like scissors.
- It is important to keep the inner thighs contracted the entire time.

· sets and reps ·		
BEGINNER	1 set	10 to 12 reps
INTERMEDIATE	2 sets	12 to 15 reps
ADVANCED	3 sets	15 to 20 reps

exercise recipe #30

towel squats

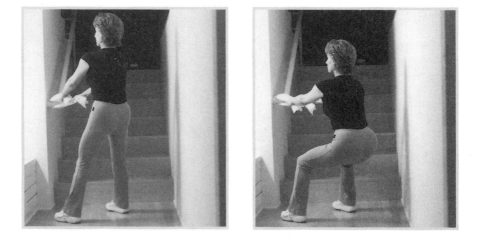

target: front of legs and buttocks
(quadriceps and gluteals)

Towel Squats are a fantastic multijointed warm-up exercise that can be done anyplace, anytime—at work, at home, on the road.

FORM

- Wrap a hand towel around a *stationary* object, such as a doorknob, banister, or post. Important: Make certain the object is tightly secured, or you could hurt yourself or break it!
- Grab each end of the towel with your hands.
- Pull away from the towel so your arms are straight and you feel as if the towel were an extension of your arms.
- Place your feet hip-distance apart.
- Feet are parallel and pointed straight in front of you.
- Your back is straight. Do not slouch.

- Contract your abs.
- Keep your shoulders and upper neck relaxed, your head facing forward.

TECHNIQUE

- Squat down slowly as if your buttocks were going to land in a chair.
- As you drop into the squat, make sure your knees *do not go out over your toes.*
- Do not drop down deeper than the position where your thighs are parallel to the floor.
- Squeeze the buttocks as you move into and come up from the squat.
- You will feel a contraction in the front of the thighs (quads) as well.
- Do not stop the flow of movement between reps.

· sets and reps ·		
BEGINNER	1 set	10 to 12 reps
INTERMEDIATE	2 sets	12 to 15 reps
ADVANCED	3 sets	15 to 20 reps

standing leg curls

target: back of legs (hamstrings)

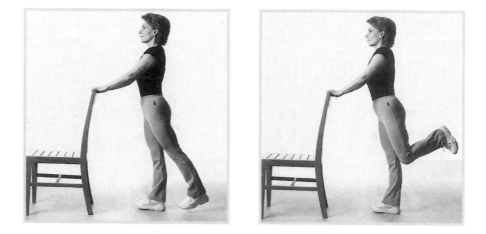

Standing Leg Curls target the three muscles in the back of your leg—the hamstring group—which are the primary movers in knee flexion. You have the option to do these without weights, or you can use ankle weights to create added resistance.

FORM

• Stand holding on to the back of a chair or counter for support, or with your hands placed on a wall. If you are leaning against a wall, place your hands shoulder-width apart and your feet about two feet from the wall.
• Contract the abdominals.
• Keep hips parallel, making sure one isn't out in front of the other.
• Maintain a neutral spine, and do not elevate the shoulders or strain your neck.

TECHNIQUE

- Lift the first foot off the ground and *slowly* bring the heel of the foot straight back toward your buttocks.
- As you lift your foot upward, you contract the muscles in the back of the leg.
- Bring your foot as close to your buttocks as possible.
- The release is very important: Do not let your foot just fall back to the ground.
- As you return the foot to the starting position, use the muscles of the back of the leg to *resist gravity*. This is the lengthening action.
- Do not *rest* or *stop the foot* on the ground but immediately start back up again to perform the next repetition.

· sets and reps (per leg) ·

BEGINNER	1 set	5 to 10 reps
INTERMEDIATE	2 sets	10 to 12 reps
ADVANCED	3 sets	12 to 15 reps

exercise recipe #32

push-ups

target: chest, arms, back, and core

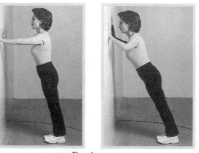

Beginner

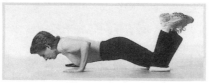

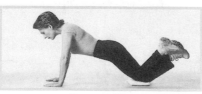

Intermediate

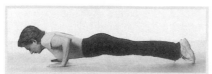

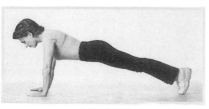

Advanced

Push-Ups are one of the best upper-body strengthening exercises you can do, and *you can do them*! There are three different levels of push-ups:

- Beginner/Easy
- Intermediate/Moderate
- Advanced/Hard

FORM FOR ALL LEVELS

- Keep your abdominals contracted the entire time.
- Always maintain a neutral spine: your head in line with your back.
- Lead with your chest and not with your chin.
- Maintain straight posture and good form.

TECHNIQUE

- *Beginner/Easy* Push-Ups can be done by placing your hands against a wall. You can also use an exercise ball. Place hands shoulder-width apart and feet hip-width apart. As you push toward the wall or the ball, you will feel the contraction across your chest and in your biceps as well. Lean in slowly and push back slowly, keeping a slight bend in your elbows. Do not drop your head or chin down.

• *Intermediate/Moderate* Push-Ups are done on the floor. Kneeling, place your hands on the floor where they will be about an inch above your shoulders and a little wider than shoulder-width apart. Cross your feet at your ankles. (Place a mat or towel under your knees to cushion and protect them.) Leading with your chest, try to come down as close to the ground as possible. Then slowly push back up, keeping a slight bend in your elbows. Abdominals stay contracted the entire time; also, keep your head in line with your spine.

• *Advanced/Hard* Push-Ups (full-out military Push-Ups) are done with your legs straight out behind you. Your hands are placed directly underneath your shoulders and you are on your toes. Your eyes are staring down at the ground. Lower your body to the floor, trying to place your chest as close to the ground as possible. Do not sink into the Push-Up or allow your body to curve or hyperextend out of plank (straight body) position. Slowly push back up to the starting position and begin the next repetition.

· sets and reps ·

BEGINNER	1 set	1 to 5 reps
INTERMEDIATE	2 sets	5 to 10 reps
ADVANCED	3 sets	10-plus reps

exercise recipe #33

lateral drops

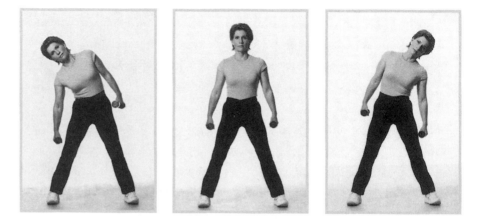

target: waist (external and internal obliques)

This simple waist exercise works the internal and external obliques, a muscle in the front of the chest called the serratus anterior, and the lower back (lumbar) muscles.

FORM

- Stand with your feet firmly planted on the ground, placed about an inch wider than shoulder-width apart.
- Maintain a slight bend in the knees.
- Abdominals are contracted and you are pulling up straight out of your hips, ribs open wide, shoulders back.
- Buttocks are squeezed tightly, so your entire lower body provides a strong, firm base.

TECHNIQUE

- Either with or without dumbbells in your hands, slowly drop to one side.
- Bring your hand as far down the side of your leg as possible.
- Maintain a straight spine the entire time and do not let your chest sink or shoulders drop.
- Your head is facing forward, eyes focused straight ahead.
- Perform the Lateral Drop slowly, feeling the contraction in your core, and start back up again slowly.
- Immediately begin to drop to the other side.

· sets and reps ·		
BEGINNER	3 sets	5 to 10 reps
INTERMEDIATE	3 sets	10 to 15 reps
ADVANCED	3 sets	15 to 20 reps

exercise recipe #34

exercise recipe #35

side leg lifts

target: outer thigh, inner thigh, and buttocks (adductors and gluteals)

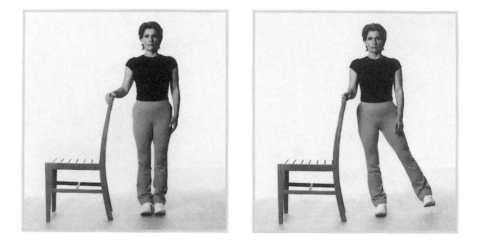

Side Leg Lifts work your gluteus medius (the upper buttocks) and the muscles of the hip that run along the outside part of your leg and the inner thighs.

FORM

- If you have good balance, you can do this without support. If not, hold on to the back of a chair, a counter, or any stationary object for support.
- Tightly contract the abdominal muscles.
- Keep your hips aligned with one another; don't allow one to come out in front of the other.
- Stand tall, with shoulders back, chest open, back straight.

TECHNIQUE

• Draw one foot away from the other, out to the side. Your foot should be flexed, toes pointed upward.

• Bring the foot as far to the side as your hip range of motion allows.

• Contract the buttocks the entire time.

• Feel the work on the side of the leg as well as at the side of the buttocks.

• Keeping your foot flexed, start slowly returning your foot to the starting position, scissoring in, this time leading with the inner thigh.

• When your working foot returns to base, do not stop or let it touch the ground, but immediately perform the next repetition.

· sets and reps (per leg) ·		
BEGINNER	3 sets	5 to 10 reps
INTERMEDIATE	3 sets	10 to 15 reps
ADVANCED	3 sets	15 to 20 reps

exercise recipe #35

· about the thirty-day design ·

I created the "30 Days" menu based on nearly two decades of writing exercise prescriptions for hundreds of patients and clients. Just as with the women I work with privately, I designed the Smart Girls dumbbell program specifically to ensure the following:

1. *Results*—by training different muscle groups each day and using a variety of exercises to stimulate muscle response and growth.

2. *Adherence*—by providing a diversity of exercises for each muscle group to avoid boredom and exercise burnout.

3. *Enjoyment*—by offering program flexibility, including "light days," every seventh day to revive body and spirit and eliminate feelings of "exercise guilt."

Think of the Exercise Recipes as your personal coach. In the beginning, you may want to review them frequently until you feel you've mastered the form and technique. After that, review them periodically just to make certain you're maintaining the integrity of your moves.

The Dumbbell Exercise Recipes and Dumbbell-Free Exercise Recipes are found on pages 116–185. They appear on the Exercise Menu under the recipe column by their numerals only.

The Stretch Recipes appear on pages 64–70 and are indicated by the letter *S* and their numeral.

The Abdominal Recipes appear on pages 82–87 and are indicated by the letters *Ab* followed by the numeral.

Muscle is magic. While you're building it you're building a life of strength, stamina, health, and pride. I've said this before, but I'm not the sole advocate of this body-building, life-altering tissue. Natalie Angier, the Pulitzer prize–winning science writer, says in her book *Woman: An Intimate Geography,* "The body needs its muscle, especially as it ages. Yet the perverse reality is that in the absence of a concerted effort to remain strong, the aging body loses muscle and gains fat."

30 Days and You're on Your Way! The beginning is not a day of the week. It's a day of the *self.* And, whatever that day is for you, when that moment strikes, it is the day you are ready to take command of your body and your health.

"30 days and you're on your way"
exercise menu

· day 1 ·

BODY PART	EXERCISE	RECIPE
Front of arms	Classic Forward Curls	#6
Back of arms	V-Backs	#5
Chest	Bench Presses	#16
Back	Kneeling One-Arm Rows	#21
Shoulders	Side Raises	#11
Upper abdominals	Traditional Crunches	Ab #4
Today's stretch	Head and Neck Rotations	S #4
	Shoulder Rolls	S #5

· day 2 ·

BODY PART	EXERCISE	RECIPE
Front of legs	Forward Lunges	#23
Back of legs	Deadlifts	#27
Front of legs and buttocks	Towel Squats	#31
Calves	Bilateral Heel Raises	#28

BODY PART	EXERCISE	RECIPE
Lower abdominals	Reverse Leg Lifts	Ab #2
Today's stretch	Hamstring Hug	S #1
	Lumbar Twist	S #2

· day 3 ·

BODY PART	EXERCISE	RECIPE
Front of arms	Hammer Curls	#8
Back of arms	Two-Arm Overhead Extensions	#2
Chest	Bench Flyes	#17
Back	Standing Bent-Over Rows	#20
Shoulders	Military Presses	#12
Obliques	Torso Twists	Ab #3
Today's stretch	Lateral Waist Bends	S #3

· day 4 ·

BODY PART	EXERCISE	RECIPE
Front of legs and buttocks	Front Squats	#22
Back of legs	Standing Leg Curls	#32
Inner thighs	Plié Squats	#30
Calves	Unilateral Heel Raises	#29

· day 4 (continued) ·

BODY PART	EXERCISE	RECIPE
Lower abdominals	Pelvic Tilts	Ab #6
Today's stretch	Seated Inner Thigh	S #6

· day 5 ·

BODY PART	EXERCISE	RECIPE
Front of arms	Supinated Curls	#7
Back of arms	One-Arm Overhead Extensions	#1
Chest	Seated Forward Flyes	#19
Back	Kneeling One-Arm Rows	#21
Back of shoulders	Reverse Flyes	#15
Core abdominals	Isometric Contractions	Ab #1
Today's stretch	Piriformis Stretch	S #7

· day 6 ·
compound lower body day

BODY PART	EXERCISE	RECIPE
Lower abdominals	Reverse Leg Lifts	Ab #2
Obliques	Torso Twists	Ab #3
Upper abdominals	Traditional Crunches	Ab #4

BODY PART	EXERCISE	RECIPE
Front of legs and buttocks	Towel Squats*	#31
Waist	Lateral Drops*	#34
Front of legs and buttocks	Forward Lunges (Right Leg)*	#23
Front of legs and buttocks	Forward Lunges (Left Leg)*	#23
Back of legs and lower back	Deadlifts	#27
Inner thighs	Plié Squats	#30
Today's stretch	Hamstring Hug	S #1

*Compound sets: Do one type of exercise followed by a different exercise, changing back and forth from one to the other until you've finished the set. For instance, you would do a set of Towel Squats and then a set of Lateral Drops, followed by the next set of Towel Squats with Lateral Drops, and so forth.

· day 7 (a take-it-easy day) ·
something is better than nothing

Abdominals	Your choice of any three	
Stretches	Your choice of any four	
Breathing and meditation		

· day 8 ·

BODY PART	EXERCISE	RECIPE
Front of arms	Seated One-Arm Biceps Curls	#9
Back of arms	Bent-Over Kickbacks	#4
Chest	Seated Forward Presses	#18
Back	Standing Bent-Over Rows	#20
Shoulders	Upright Rows	#13
Lower and upper abdominals	Combo Crunches	Ab #5
Today's stretch	Lateral Waist Bends	S #3

· day 9 ·

BODY PART	EXERCISE	RECIPE
Front of legs and buttocks	Reverse Lunges	#26
Back of legs	Standing Leg Curls	#32
Front of legs and buttocks	Towel Squats	#31
Calves	Bilateral Heel Raises	#28
Lower abdominals	Reverse Leg Lifts	Ab #2
Today's stretch	Seated Inner Thigh	S #6

· day 10 ·

BODY PART	EXERCISE	RECIPE
Front of arms	Combination Biceps Curls	#10
Back of arms	Standing Kickbacks	#3
Chest	Bench Flyes	#17
Back	Kneeling One-Arm Rows	#21
Shoulders	Single-Arm Front Lifts	#14
Lower abdominals	Pelvic Tilts	Ab #6
Today's stretch	Lumbar Twist	S #2

· day 11 ·

BODY PART	EXERCISE	RECIPE
Front of legs and buttocks	Walking Lunges	#25
Back of legs and lower back	Deadlifts	#27
Front of legs and buttocks	Towel Squats	#31
Calves	Unilateral Heel Raises	#29
Obliques	Torso Twists	Ab #3
Today's stretch	Piriformis Stretch	S #7

· day 12 ·

BODY PART	EXERCISE	RECIPE
Front of arms	Classic Forward Curls	#6
Back of arms	Bent-Over Kickbacks	#4
Chest	Bench Presses	#16
Back	Standing Bent-Over Rows	#20
Shoulders	Military Presses	#12
Upper abdominals	Traditional Crunches	Ab #4
Today's stretch	Head and Neck Rotations	S #4
	Shoulder Rolls	S #5

· day 13 ·
compound lower-body day

BODY PART	EXERCISE	RECIPE
Lower abdominals	Reverse Leg Lifts	Ab #2
Obliques	Torso Twists	Ab #3
Upper abdominals	Traditional Crunches	Ab #4
Front of legs and buttocks	Towel Squats*	#31
Outer/inner thighs and buttocks	Side Leg Lifts*	#35
Front of legs and buttocks	Forward Lunges (Right Leg)*	#23
Front of legs and buttocks	Forward Lunges (Left Leg)*	#23

BODY PART	EXERCISE	RECIPE
Back of legs and lower back	Deadlifts	#27
Inner thighs	Plié Squats	#30
Today's stretch	Lumbar Twist	S #2

* Compound sets.

· day 14 (a take-it-easy day) ·
tide me over

Push-Ups (#33)

Three of your favorite Ab Flatteners

Three stretches

Deep breathing

Five minutes of meditation or relaxation

· day 15 ·

BODY PART	EXERCISE	RECIPE
Front of legs and buttocks	Reverse Lunges	#26
Back of legs	Standing Leg Curls	#32
Inner thighs	Plié Squats	#30
Calves	Bilateral Heel Raises	#28
Core	Isometric Contractions	Ab #1
Today's stretch	Lateral Waist Bends	S #3

· day 16 ·

BODY PART	EXERCISE	RECIPE
Front of arms	Seated One-Arm Biceps Curls	#9
Back of arms	One-Arm Overhead Extensions	#1
Chest	Seated Forward Presses	#18
Back	Standing Bent-Over Rows	#20
Front of shoulders	Upright Rows	#13
Lower abdominals	Pelvic Tilts	Ab #6
Today's stretch	Piriformis Stretch	S #7

· day 17 ·

BODY PART	EXERCISE	RECIPE
Front of legs	Forward Lunges Using Step or Stool	#24
Back of legs and lower back	Deadlifts	#27
Front of legs and buttocks	Towel Squats	#31
Calves	Unilateral Heel Raises	#29
Obliques	Torso Twists	Ab #3
Today's stretch	Lumbar Twist	S #2

· day 18 ·

BODY PART	EXERCISE	RECIPE
Front of arms	Combination Biceps Curls	#10
Back of arms	Bent-Over Kickbacks	#4
Chest	Seated Forward Flyes	#19
Back	Kneeling One-Arm Rows	#21
Shoulders	Single-Arm Front Lifts	#14
Lower abdominals	Pelvic Tilts	Ab #6
Today's stretch	Lateral Waist Bends	S #3

· day 19 ·

BODY PART	EXERCISE	RECIPE
Front of legs and buttocks	Forward Lunges	#23
Outer/inner thighs and buttocks	Side Leg Lifts	#35
Inner thighs	Plié Squats	#30
Calves	Unilateral Heel Raises	#29
Lower abdominals	Reverse Leg Lifts	Ab #2
Today's stretch	Hamstring Hug	S #1

· day 20 ·
compound arm day

BODY PART	EXERCISE	RECIPE
Lower abdominals	Pelvic Tilts	Ab #6
Obliques	Torso Twists	Ab #3
Upper abdominals	Traditional Crunches	Ab #4
Front of arms	Classic Forward Curls*	#6
Back of arms	Standing Kickbacks*	#3
Shoulders	Side Raises*	#11
Waist	Lateral Drops*	#34
Chest	Push-Ups*	#33
Back	Standing Bent-Over Rows*	#20
Today's stretch	Seated Inner Thigh	S #6

*Compound sets.

· day 21 (a take-it-easy day) ·
a little goes a long way

Lateral Waist Bends (S #3)

Lumbar Twist (S #2)

Hamstring Hug (S #1)

Pelvic Tilts (Ab #6)

Five minutes of quiet time

· day 22 ·

BODY PART	EXERCISE	RECIPE
Front of legs and buttocks	Forward Lunges Using Step or Stool	#24
Back of legs	Standing Leg Curls	#32
Inner thighs	Plié Squats	#30
Calves	Bilateral Heel Raises	#28
Lower abdominals	Reverse Leg Lifts	Ab #2
Today's stretch	Piriformis Stretch	S #7

· day 23 ·

BODY PART	EXERCISE	RECIPE
Front of arms	Hammer Curls	#8
Back of arms	V-Backs	#5
Chest	Bench Presses	#16
Back	Kneeling One-Arm Rows	#21
Shoulders	Side Raises	#11
Upper abdominals	Traditional Crunches	Ab #4
Today's stretch	Hamstring Hug	S #1

· day 24 ·

BODY PART	EXERCISE	RECIPE
Front of legs and buttocks	Walking Lunges	#25
Back of legs	Standing Leg Curls	#32
Inner thighs	Plié Squats	#30
Calves	Unilateral Heel Raises	#29
Lower abdominals	Pelvic Tilts	Ab #6
Today's stretch	Lumbar Twist	S #2

· day 25 ·

BODY PART	EXERCISE	RECIPE
Front of arms	Supinated Curls	#7
Back of arms	V-Backs	#5
Chest	Push-Ups	#33
Back	Standing Bent-Over Rows	#20
Shoulders	Military Presses	#12
Obliques	Torso Twists	Ab #3
Today's stretch	Head and Neck Rotations	S #4
	Shoulder Rolls	S #5

· day 26 ·

BODY PART	EXERCISE	RECIPE
Front of legs and buttocks	Front Squats	#22
Back of legs	Standing Leg Curls	#32
Inner thighs	Plié Squats	#30
Calves	Unilateral Heel Raises	#29
Lower abdominals	Reverse Leg Lifts	Ab #2
Today's stretch	Seated Inner Thigh	S #6

· day 27 ·
compound arm set

BODY PART	EXERCISE	RECIPE
Lower and upper abdominals	Combo Crunches	Ab #5
Obliques	Torso Twists	Ab #3
Upper abdominals	Traditional Crunches	Ab #4
Chest*	Bench Flyes*	#17
Back of arms*	Two-Arm Overhead Extensions*	#2
Back*	Kneeling One-Arm Rows*	#21
Front of arms*	Supinated Curls*	#7
Shoulders	Upright Rows	#13
Today's stretches	Lateral Waist Bends	S #3
	Hamstring Hug	S #1

*Compound sets.

· day 28 (a take-it-easy day) ·
working my favorite parts

Any three of your favorite Smart Girls dumbbell exercises
Any two of your favorite Smart Girls abdominal exercises
Five minutes of deep breathing and relaxation
One affirmation about how great you are doing!

· day 29 ·

BODY PART	EXERCISE	RECIPE
Front of legs and buttocks	Forward Lunges Using Step or Stool	#24
Back of legs and lower back	Deadlifts	#27
Front of legs and buttocks	Towel Squats	#31
Calves	Bilateral Heel Raises	#28
Upper abdominals	Traditional Crunches	Ab #4
Today's stretch	Piriformis Stretch	S #7

· day 30 ·

BODY PART	EXERCISE	RECIPE
Front of arms	Combination Biceps Curls	#10
Back of arms	Standing Kickbacks	#3

BODY PART	EXERCISE	RECIPE
Chest	Seated Forward Presses	#18
Back	Standing Bent-Over Rows	#20
Back of shoulders	Reverse Flyes	#15
Core abdominals	Isometric Contractions	Ab #1
Today's stretch	Lumbar Twist	S #2

· 11 ·

smart girls ask
smart questions

SAMANTHA, a twenty-six-year-old group sales manager from Maryland, asks:

I really like the Smart Girls dumbbell program because I want the look of lean muscles. But I am also concerned with burning the maximum calories I can during my workouts. Am I burning as many calories lifting dumbbells as I would be doing aerobics?

JUDITH: No, you are not burning as many "active" calories doing thirty minutes of your Smart Girls dumbbell exercises as you are while doing thirty minutes of aerobics. However, and this is a mighty important however, the more muscle you have the more passive calories you burn because, as I wrote in chapter 1, a body rich in muscle burns more calories at rest. In the American College of Sports Medicine Guidelines for Exercise Testing and Prescription, it states, "Both aerobic exercise and resistance training can contribute to the loss of body weight and fat stores and maximize the potential to maintain these changes." I have created the "How Much Do I Burn?" chart (located in the appendix) that is a great tool to give you an estimate of the amount of calories you will burn doing your Smart Girls exercises for thirty minutes. Locate your weight and beneath it find the approximate number of calories you will burn. I've also included the caloric expenditure of other popular activities on the chart, which I think you will find useful.

ELLEN,   an artist and community activist, is very proactive when it comes to her diet and exercise.

I spend an awful lot of time talking about calories, counting calories, burning calories, but to tell you the truth, I don't know exactly what a calorie is.

JUDITH: In its simplest terms, a calorie is a unit of heat. In human nutrition, a calorie—more correctly called a kilocalorie (kcal)—is defined as the *amount of heat necessary to raise the temperature of 1 kilogram (1 liter) of water 1 degree C, from 14.5 to 15.5 C.* For instance, if your favorite dessert is 200 kcals, then the energy captured inside the chemical bonds of the dessert, if liberated, would change the temperature of 200 liters of water by 1 degree C. A Big Mac has a caloric value of 570 kcal and would contain the equivalent heat energy to increase the temperature of 570 liters of water 1 degree C.

WENDY   is a special investigator for the U.S. Department of Justice.

What exactly does BMR mean and why is it important for my diet and exercise programming?

JUDITH: BMR stands for your Basal Metabolic Rate, also called your resting metabolic rate. It is the minimum level of energy needed to keep your body functioning while you are awake. It is a valuable measurement to help you design your nutrition program. It has been estimated that your

BMR decreases about 2 percent per decade primarily due to loss of fat-free mass (muscle). It has also been estimated that women's resting metabolism is about 5 to 10 percent lower than men's. Men are stronger not because their muscle is different from women's, they just have more of it. Genetically, women just carry more fat than men (sorry about that). Fat is metabolically less active than muscle. More good reasons for you to use dumbbells.

CAROLE,   a manager of commercial properties, is in her early fifties. She is an avid and accomplished tennis player who also works out regularly at the gym.
When I use the stair stepper at my gym, in addition to the number of calories I'm burning, it gives me a METs reading. What does that mean?

JUDITH: METs are multiples of your BMR or the amount of oxygen you consume at rest. One MET is about 3.6 milliliters of oxygen per kilogram of body weight per minute. What this means is that a 120-pound woman at rest uses approximately 200 milliliters of oxygen per minute. An exercise load at 2 METs uses twice your resting metabolism (or about 400 milliliters of oxygen per minute), and an exercise load at 3 METs uses three times the resting energy expenditure. Take a look at the following list and I think it will help you better understand how METs translate to the intensity of your physical activity.

Obviously billiards is not an especially vigorous activity but look how challenging cross-country skiing and running can be! Commercial exercise equipment often inflates the MET value of its activity—the equipment's computer is programmed to rate its activity with a higher MET value than warranted. So it registers you are burning a higher number of calories than you actually are. (Usually those

ACTIVITY	MET LEVEL RANGE
Billiards	2.5
Croquet	3.6
Cross-country skiing	6–12+
Cycling	3–8+
Tennis	4–9+
Swimming	4–8+
Running	8.7–16.3
Playing music	2–3
Roller or ice skating	5–8

machines are the most popular in the gym.) The list above gives you a reality check. If you are on a stair climber or elliptical machine and it gives a MET of 9, ask yourself, "Am I working as hard as I would be if I were running?" If the answer is no, then just be aware that your caloric expenditure is not really as high as you think it is.

JOANNA,   a professional dancer and singer in her late twenties, has toured the United States in the road companies of *Mamma Mia*.

I am hearing more and more in the media about Body Mass Index. Is this the same as your body composition?

JUDITH: The *Body Mass Index* (also called Quetelet's index) assesses weight relative to height. It is nonspecific: It does not take into consideration gender, age, or your percentage of body fat versus lean mass. It is used mainly in epidemiological studies and by health organizations to give generalized guidelines for disease risk and obesity. If you want to find out your BMI, refer to the chart in the appendix. Locate your height, which is given in inches, and your weight. The number at the top of the column will be your BMI.

Body composition is the ratio of body fat to lean body mass; it is a measurement *specific to your own body*. There are several different techniques to measure body composition. Following is a brief description of five of the most frequently used and most reliable methods.

HYDROSTATIC (UNDERWATER) WEIGHING: This is considered the gold standard in measuring body composition. It is based on the principles discovered by the Greek mathematical genius Archimedes. As the story goes, King Hiero had ordered a gold crown to be made by a new crown maker. When it was delivered, even though it weighed what it was supposed to, the king suspected the goldsmith of cheating him out of the gold provided to him to make the crown. He called in Archimedes, the leading mathematician and research scientist of the day, to investigate the crown's composition. Had the gold been adulterated with another metal, such as silver? Archimedes pondered the problem for some time until one day, during the simple ritual of taking a bath, he came upon the methodology for researching this problem. He noticed that as he dropped down into his bath, the water overflowed in relation to his body's density. He knew gold was denser than silver. He then determined he could calculate the crown's density by submerging it in water to resolve the mystery. As it turned out, the king's suspicions were justified. The crown maker had not used pure gold, but had added silver to the amalgam. (My guess is, although I have no proof, the crown maker ended up being lion feed.)

The Archimedes Principle, as it is called, is the basis of hydrostatic weighing. Your percentage of body fat is computed from your body density (the ratio of body mass to body volume). Although hydrostatic weighing is considered the most accurate by most exercise physiologists and research scientists, certain factors have to be taken into consideration, including residual lung volume. It is also the most stressful and cumbersome of the measurement techniques and might be contraindicated for people who are apprehensive about being submerged in water.

CALIPERS: Calipers are used to determine your percentage of body fat through skinfold measurements. The skinfolds may be taken at the abdomen, triceps, biceps, chest, calf, back, and the top of the thigh. The theory behind calipers is that the amount of subcutaneous fat (fat underneath the skin) at the various sites correlates to the amount of total body fat. Caliper measurements can be very accurate, providing a skilled technician takes the measurements.

WAIST TO HIP RATIO (WHR): This is a very simple way of measuring body composition and estimating health risks related to obesity. The WHR measurement is the circumference of the waist divided by the circumference of the hips. For instance, if your waist is 27 inches and your hips are 37 you would divide 27 by 37, and your WHR would be 0.73.

Women's WHR should be below 0.82
Men's WHR should be below 0.94

The pattern of body fat distribution is a valuable predictor of health-related problems. Trunk or abdominal fat is directly correlated to increased risk for type 2 diabetes, elevated blood lipids, high blood pressure, and heart disease.

BIOELECTRICAL IMPEDANCE ANALYSIS (BIA): This is a very accurate, noninvasive, easy-to-administer technique to measure body composition in a clinical or fitness setting. The

BIA meter is about the size of a laptop computer. It measures water in the muscle by passing a painless, low-voltage current through the tissue. Muscle is around 70 to 75 percent water. Water is a good conductor of electrical current. Fat is not. The speed with which the current flows through the muscle measures the fat-free mass and inversely gives a reading of the body fat percentage. If you are going to have a BIA test to measure your body composition, make sure you prepare in the following ways:

- Do not eat or drink for four hours before your test.
- Avoid moderate or vigorous activity for twelve hours before testing.
- Do not drink alcohol for forty-eight hours.
- Avoid taking diuretic agents, unless prescribed by your physician, and avoid caffeine drinks, including soda, for four hours.

DUAL ENERGY X-RAY ABSORPTIOMETRY SCAN (DEXA): This is a full body scan that takes around ten minutes and uses low-energy X rays that pass through bone, fat, and lean tissue. In addition to evaluating percentage of body fat, DEXAs are most commonly used to measure bone density and determine if there is any bone loss that could lead to osteoporosis. DEXA machines are mainly found in clinical settings and is a fairly expensive diagnostic method by which to test body composition alone.

ALISON is a thirty-year-old entrepreneur who studied dance for most of her life and doesn't have a lot of extra time these days between running her business and getting her master's degree.

The Smart Girls dumbbell program workout is ideal for me because I have so little time these days for fitness. I know working with dumbbells is not "aerobic" exercise but can you explain to me the difference between "aerobic" and "anaerobic" exercise?

JUDITH: Anaerobic exercise utilizes energy already stored inside the cells. The types of exercises classified as anaerobic are limited to short bursts of vigorous activity, for example, a tennis serve, golf swing, power lift, or sprint.

Aerobic exercise, such as endurance exercises like marathon running, long-distance jogging, and swimming, requires increases in a steady rate of oxygen, a response to increasing your heart rate, so the cells can break down the molecules (glucose) to provide the body with the energy necessary to sustain the exercise over a long period of time.

TRISHA,   thirty-three, came to see me during her first trimester of pregnancy. She was concerned about doing everything possible to protect her health and the health of her baby. *Is it safe for me to use dumbbells during my pregnancy?*

JUDITH: This depends on the consent of your physician and the status of your health during your pregnancy. "Don't start any new exercise you haven't done before," advises Dr. Philip Brooks, a renowned obstetrician and gynecologist in private practice in Beverly Hills, California, a clinical professor at the David Geffen School of Medicine at UCLA, and one of the country's leading authorities on gynecologic laparoscopic surgery. "There are no risks engendered by lifting dumbbells during pregnancy itself, if you were doing it before you got pregnant," says Dr. Brooks. "However, it is not a good idea to take it up for the first time while you are pregnant." The reason for this, he explains, is that "the lifting action increases blood flow to tissues and muscle, creating swelling which could result in some physical discomfort. Because pregnancy itself, with all the natural changes taking place in the body, can be an uncomfortable situation for many women, it is not a good idea to introduce anything new that would cause additional pain." But Dr. Brooks does believe pregnant women benefit from exercise if they participate in a sensible program. "Exercise helps preserve muscle tone and protect the back from the discomfort of lumbar lordosis (swayback), which is caused by the natural forward shift in body gravity during pregnancy." And, Dr. Brooks offers one other encouraging note about exercising during pregnancy: "It may even help a woman return to her prepregnancy figure faster."

KATE   is a writer in her late forties who travels frequently throughout the world.
I have heard that if you exercise enough, you don't need to diet. Is this true?

JUDITH: This is one of those complicated half "yes," half "no" answers with a little "maybe" thrown in. In order to clarify, we need to break down the numbers. One pound of stored fat equals 3,500 calories. If you want to lose one pound a week, you would have to create a caloric deficit of 3,500 calories, or 500 a day. You have three options in order to create this deficit:

1. You can reduce your energy intake by 500 calories (how much you eat).
2. You can increase your energy output by 500 calories (how much you exercise).
3. You can do a combination of both!

Let's refer again to the "How Much Do I Burn?" chart in the appendix: If you weigh 135 pounds and you perform medium-intensity aerobic activity for thirty minutes you will burn approximately 190 calories. In order for you to reach your 500-calorie-a-day goal, you would have to perform your aerobic activity for around 90 minutes. Can it be done? You bet—if you have an hour and a half you can spend on the treadmill or taking a vigorous walk each day. Most people don't have that time flexibility or tolerance for exercise. You can also reduce your energy intake by 500 calories, which is also difficult to do.

And that is how the popular and most successful weight management formula of all time developed:

diet + exercise = the most realistic program for *weight loss*

I wish I could be by your side as you begin your strength-altering, life-enhancing journey. It is an important endeavor, one which will change you both physically and emotionally. And one, I believe, you will never regret. Congratulations on giving yourself the gifts of fitness and good health!

If you have any questions regarding your dumbbell workouts or exercise, you may e-mail me directly at: **judith@smartgirlsdodumbbells.com**

appendix

· 6-site body evaluation log ·

date: _____

MEASUREMENTS	CURRENT	GOAL	DO YOU BELIEVE THIS IS ATTAINABLE?	WHY?
Weight				
Bust				
Waist				
Hips				
Upper Arms				
Upper Thighs				
Calves				

Instructions for taking accurate measurements:

1. Stand erect, but relax limbs being measured.
2. Wrap tape measure around the area being measured *without* pinching the skin.
3. Take hip and upper thigh measurements around the widest part.
4. Measure the upper arm midway between the elbow and the shoulder.
5. Measure waist at the narrowest part, above the belly button and below the breastbone.

· daily dumbbell workout schedule ·
date: _____

MUSCLE GROUP	EXERCISE	SETS	REPS	WEIGHTS	FEELINGS OF ENERGY EXPENDED

Notes for next workout:

· "feelings of energy expended" scale ·				
3–4	5–6	7–8	9–10	11–12
AVERAGE	GOOD	VERY GOOD	ALMOST PERFECT	EXEMPLARY

The "Feelings of Energy Expended" scale is designed to help you monitor your dumbbell workout. After you have completed your dumbbell set, ask yourself, "On a scale of 3 to 12, how do I feel about the quality of my effort? Was I working with concentration or passivity? Was I visualizing my muscles working or was I distracted? Was I working with integrity or was I a little sloppy?" It is not about how difficult the work feels, but about *how you feel* about the effort you are applying.

· how much do i burn? ·

The chart below gives you the approximate amount of kilocalories (kcals) you burn in thirty minutes performing various exercises and activities. For example, if you weigh 120 pounds and you're doing medium-intensity aerobics, you will burn about 169 kcals for your thirty minutes of exercise.

BODY WEIGHT (in Pounds)	100	105	110	115	120	125	130	135	140	145	150	155	160	165
Doing Dumbbells	117	123	129	134	141	147	152	158	164	170	176	182	188	194
Aerobics, Medium-Intensity	140	147	154	162	169	176	183	190	197	204	211	218	225	232
Aerobics, High-Intensity	184	193	202	212	221	230	239	249	258	267	276	285	295	304
Cycling Outdoors	136	143	150	157	164	170	177	184	191	198	205	211	218	225
Stationary Bike	87	91	96	100	105	109	113	117	122	127	131	135	140	144
Jogging	184	193	203	212	221	230	239	249	258	267	276	285	295	304
Jumping Rope	220	231	243	254	266	276	287	298	309	320	331	342	353	365
Swimming	212	223	234	244	255	266	277	287	298	308	319	330	340	351
Tennis	148	156	163	171	178	186	193	201	208	216	223	230	238	245
Walking	117	123	129	135	141	147	152	158	164	170	177	182	188	195
Water Aerobics	90	94.5	99	104	108	113	117	122	126	131	135	140	144	149
Yoga/Pilates	90	94.5	99	104	108	113	117	122	126	131	135	140	144	149
BODY WEIGHT (in Pounds)	170	175	180	185	190	195	200	205	210	215	220	225	230	235
Doing Dumbbells	199	205	211	217	223	229	235	240	246	252	258	264	270	276
Aerobics, Medium-Intensity	239	246	253	260	267	274	281	288	295	302	309	316	323	330
Aerobics, High-Intensity	313	322	331	341	350	359	368	377	387	396	405	414	423	433
Cycling Outdoors	232	239	245	252	259	266	273	280	286	293	300	307	314	320
Stationary Bike	148	153	157	161	166	170	175	179	183	188	192	196	201	205
Jogging	313	322	331	341	350	359	368	377	387	396	405	414	423	433
Jumping Rope	376	387	398	409	420	431	442	453	464	475	486	497	509	519
Swimming	362	372	383	394	404	415	425	436	447	457	468	479	489	450
Tennis	253	260	268	275	282	290	297	305	312	320	327	334	342	350
Walking	199	205	211	217	223	229	235	240	246	252	258	264	270	276
Water Aerobics	153	158	162	167	171	176	180	185	189	194	198	203	207	212
Yoga/Pilates	153	158	162	167	171	176	180	185	189	194	198	203	207	212

· what is your body mass index? ·

To find your BMI, locate your height in the left-hand column and your weight in the grid. Your BMI is listed at the top.

	19	20	21	22	23	24	25	26	27	28	29	30	31	32	33	34	35
HEIGHT (Inches)							BODY WEIGHT (Pounds)										
58	91	96	100	105	110	115	119	124	129	134	138	143	148	153	158	162	167
59	94	99	104	109	114	119	124	128	133	138	143	148	153	158	163	168	173
60	97	102	107	112	118	123	128	133	138	143	148	153	158	163	168	174	179
61	100	106	111	116	122	127	132	137	143	148	153	158	164	169	174	180	185
62	104	109	115	120	126	131	136	142	147	153	158	164	169	175	180	186	191
63	107	113	118	124	130	135	141	146	152	158	163	169	175	180	186	191	197
64	110	116	122	128	134	140	145	151	157	163	169	174	180	186	192	197	204
65	114	120	126	132	138	144	150	156	162	168	174	180	186	192	198	204	210
66	118	124	130	136	142	148	155	161	167	173	179	186	192	198	204	210	216
67	121	127	134	140	146	153	159	166	172	178	185	191	198	204	211	217	223
68	125	131	138	144	151	158	164	171	177	184	190	197	203	210	216	223	230
69	128	135	142	149	155	162	169	176	182	189	196	203	209	216	223	230	236
70	132	139	146	153	160	167	174	181	188	195	202	209	216	222	229	236	243
71	136	143	150	157	165	172	179	186	193	200	208	215	222	229	236	243	250
72	140	147	154	162	169	177	184	191	199	206	213	221	228	235	242	250	258
73	144	151	159	166	174	182	189	197	204	212	219	227	235	242	250	257	265
74	148	155	163	171	179	186	194	202	210	218	225	233	241	249	256	264	272
75	152	160	168	176	184	192	200	208	216	224	232	240	248	256	264	272	279
76	156	164	172	180	189	197	205	213	221	230	238	246	254	263	271	279	287

	36	37	38	39	40	41	42	43	44	45	46	47	48	49	50	51	52	53	54
HEIGHT (Inches)								BODY WEIGHT (Pounds)											
58	172	177	181	186	191	196	201	205	210	215	220	224	229	234	239	244	248	253	258
59	178	183	188	193	198	203	208	212	217	222	227	232	237	242	247	252	257	262	267
60	184	189	194	199	204	209	215	220	225	230	235	240	245	250	255	261	266	271	276
61	190	195	201	206	211	217	222	227	232	238	243	248	254	259	264	269	275	280	285
62	196	202	207	213	218	224	229	235	240	246	251	256	262	267	273	278	284	289	295
63	203	208	214	220	225	231	237	242	248	254	259	265	270	278	282	287	293	299	304
64	209	215	221	227	232	238	244	250	256	262	267	273	279	285	291	296	302	308	314
65	216	222	228	234	240	246	252	258	264	270	276	282	288	294	300	306	262	267	27
66	223	229	235	241	247	253	260	266	272	278	284	291	297	303	309	315	322	328	334
67	230	236	242	249	255	261	268	274	280	287	293	299	306	312	319	325	331	338	344
68	236	243	249	256	262	269	276	282	289	295	302	308	315	322	328	335	341	348	354
69	243	250	257	263	270	277	284	291	297	304	311	318	324	331	338	345	351	358	365
70	250	257	264	271	278	285	292	299	306	313	320	327	334	341	348	355	362	369	376
71	257	265	272	279	286	293	301	308	315	322	329	338	343	351	358	365	372	379	386
72	265	272	279	287	294	302	309	316	324	331	338	346	353	361	368	375	383	390	397
73	272	280	288	295	302	310	318	325	333	340	348	355	363	371	378	386	393	401	408
74	280	287	295	303	311	319	326	334	342	350	358	365	373	381	389	396	404	412	420
75	287	295	303	311	319	327	335	343	351	359	367	375	383	391	399	407	415	423	431
76	295	304	312	320	328	336	344	353	361	369	377	385	394	402	410	418	426	435	443

· bmi classifications ·

	BMI	OBESITY CLASSIFICATION	DISEASE RISK	
UNDERWEIGHT	< 18.5	—	—	—
NORMAL	18.5–24.9	—	—	—
OVERWEIGHT	25.0–29.9	—	Increased	High
OBESITY	30.0–34.9	I	High	Very high
OBESITY	35.0–39.9	II	Very high	Very high
EXTREME OBESITY	≥40	III	Extremely high	Extremely high